Nature's Pharmacy: Herbal Remedies for Modern-Day Illnesses

Table of Contents

- Green Tea

5. Mental Health and Emotional Well-being
   - Anxiety and Stress Relief
     - Ashwagandha
     - Valerian
     - Lemon Balm
     - Passionflower
   - Improving Sleep Quality
     - Chamomile
     - Lavender
     - Hops
     - Skullcap
   - Enhancing Cognitive Function
     - Ginkgo Biloba
     - Rosemary
     - Bacopa
     - Rhodiola

6. Women's Health
   - Menstrual Health and PMS
     - Chaste Tree Berry
     - Dong Quai
     - Raspberry Leaf
     - Evening Primrose Oil
   - Menopause Relief
     - Black Cohosh
     - Red Clover
     - Sage
     - Wild Yam
   - Reproductive Health
     - Maca Root
     - Shatavari
     - Vitex
     - Tribulus

7. Herbs for Children's Health
   - Safe Herbal Remedies for Children
   - Treating Common Childhood Ailments
     - Chamomile for Colic and Sleep
     - Fennel for Digestive Issues
     - Elderberry for Immune Support
     - Licorice Root for Coughs

8. Special Topics in Herbal Medicine
   - Herbs for Detoxification
     - Dandelion
     - Milk Thistle
     - Burdock Root
     - Cilantro
   - Enhancing Physical Performance
     - Ginseng

Introduction: The Healing Power of Herbs

For centuries, herbs have been revered for their medicinal properties, culinary uses, and ability to enhance our well-being. In an age dominated by synthetic pharmaceuticals and high-tech medical interventions, the gentle yet powerful healing properties of herbs offer a natural alternative or complement to conventional treatments. This book is a journey into the world of herbal medicine, where tradition meets modern science to provide a holistic approach to health and wellness.

From the bustling apothecaries of ancient civilizations to the modern kitchens and gardens of today, herbs have been an integral part of human history. They have played a crucial role in healing rituals, dietary practices, and cultural traditions across the globe. Each herb carries a unique profile of active compounds that interact with our bodies in intricate and beneficial ways, offering remedies for a multitude of ailments.

In this book, we will explore the rich tapestry of herbal knowledge, delving into the origins, properties, and applications of a wide variety of herbs. We will uncover the scientific principles behind their therapeutic effects, examine historical anecdotes, and provide practical guidance on how to incorporate these natural wonders into your daily life.

Whether you are a seasoned herbalist or a curious beginner, "The Healing Power of Herbs" aims to inspire and educate. By understanding and utilizing the gifts of nature, we can empower ourselves to take control of our health, enhance our well-being, and reconnect with the natural world.

Join me on this enlightening journey as we rediscover the timeless wisdom of herbs and their profound impact on our physical, emotional, and spiritual health. Together, we will unlock the secrets of these botanical treasures and embrace the healing power that lies within them.

The History of Herbal Medicine

The story of herbal medicine is as old as human civilization itself. Long before the advent of modern science and synthetic drugs, people relied on the natural world to cure their ailments, boost their immunity, and maintain their overall health. The roots of herbal medicine are deeply intertwined with the cultural, spiritual, and daily lives of our ancestors, stretching across continents and millennia.

Ancient Beginnings

The earliest evidence of medicinal plant use dates back to the Paleolithic era, around 60,000 years ago. Archaeological discoveries, such as the remains of medicinal plants in prehistoric burial sites, suggest that early humans had an intricate knowledge of their natural surroundings and used plants for therapeutic purposes. Ancient civilizations documented their herbal practices in various forms, such as clay tablets, papyrus scrolls, and carvings on temple walls.

Mesopotamia and Egypt

In Mesopotamia, the cradle of civilization, ancient texts like the "Sumerian Clay Tablets" and the "Code of Hammurabi" contain some of the earliest recorded uses of medicinal plants. The Egyptians, renowned for their advancements in medicine, documented their herbal knowledge extensively. The "Ebers Papyrus," dating back to around 1550 BCE, is one of the oldest and most comprehensive medical texts, listing hundreds of plants and their uses.

China and India

In the East, traditional Chinese medicine (TCM) and Ayurveda in India represent some of the oldest, continuously practiced systems of herbal medicine. TCM, with texts like the "Shennong Ben Cao Jing" (The Divine Farmer's Materia Medica), dating to around 200 BCE, categorizes herbs by their properties and therapeutic effects. Ayurveda, whose roots lie in the ancient Vedas written around 1500 BCE, emphasizes balance and holistic health, using herbs as a cornerstone of its practices.

Greece and Rome

The ancient Greeks and Romans furthered the knowledge of herbal medicine through scholars like Hippocrates, known as the "Father of Medicine," and Dioscorides, whose work "De Materia Medica" became a foundational text for centuries. Galen, a Roman physician, also made significant contributions, developing theories that influenced medical practices well into the Renaissance.

Medieval to Renaissance

During the medieval period, herbal knowledge was preserved and expanded upon in monasteries and by scholars in the Islamic world. The translation of classical texts into Arabic and later into Latin during the Crusades helped reintroduce this knowledge to Europe. Avicenna's "The Canon of Medicine," written in the 11th century, was a landmark work that synthesized Greek, Roman, and Islamic knowledge.

The Renaissance saw a revival of interest in botanical studies, spurred by the invention of the printing press, which allowed for the widespread dissemination of herbal texts. Herbals, books describing plants and their uses, became popular, with notable works by authors like Nicholas Culpeper and Leonhart Fuchs.

Modern Era

The advent of the scientific method in the 17th and 18th centuries brought a more systematic approach to the study of plants. The development of chemistry and pharmacology allowed scientists to isolate active compounds in herbs, leading to the creation of modern medicines. Despite the rise of synthetic drugs, the 20th century saw a resurgence of interest in herbal medicine, driven by a growing awareness of the limitations and side effects of pharmaceuticals.

Contemporary Herbal Medicine

Today, herbal medicine continues to evolve, integrating traditional wisdom with modern scientific research. Herbs are studied not only for their individual properties but also for their synergistic effects, reflecting a holistic understanding of health. The global movement towards natural and sustainable health practices has further fueled interest in herbal remedies.

As we navigate the complexities of modern health challenges, the history of herbal medicine offers valuable insights. It reminds us of our deep connection to the natural world and the timeless wisdom that plants hold. By embracing this heritage, we can continue to explore the healing power of herbs, guided by both ancient traditions and contemporary science.

The Science Behind Herbal Remedies

Herbal remedies have been used for millennia, but it is only in recent decades that modern science has begun to uncover the mechanisms behind their efficacy. The intersection of traditional knowledge and contemporary research has illuminated how herbs work at a biochemical level, providing a foundation for their continued use in modern medicine. This chapter delves into the scientific principles underlying herbal remedies, exploring the active compounds, mechanisms of action, and evidence-based benefits of these natural healers.

Active Compounds in Herbs

Herbs contain a myriad of bioactive compounds that contribute to their therapeutic effects. These compounds can be broadly categorized into several groups:

Alkaloids

Alkaloids are nitrogen-containing compounds known for their potent physiological effects. Examples include morphine from the opium poppy, which is a powerful pain reliever, and quinine from cinchona bark, historically used to treat malaria.

Flavonoids

Flavonoids are a class of polyphenolic compounds found in many plants, known for their antioxidant, anti-inflammatory, and anticancer properties. Quercetin, found in onions and apples, is a well-studied flavonoid that exhibits a range of health benefits.

Terpenes and Terpenoids

These compounds are responsible for the aromatic qualities of many herbs and have diverse medicinal properties. For instance, menthol from peppermint oil has analgesic and cooling effects, while ginkgolides from ginkgo biloba improve blood circulation and cognitive function.

Glycosides

Glycosides are compounds that yield sugars and other active substances upon hydrolysis. Cardiac glycosides, such as digoxin from foxglove, are used to treat heart conditions by increasing the force of cardiac contractions.

Tannins

Tannins are polyphenolic compounds with astringent properties, found in herbs like witch hazel and oak bark. They are used for their ability to constrict tissues and reduce bleeding.

Mechanisms of Action

The therapeutic effects of herbal remedies can be attributed to various mechanisms of action, often involving complex interactions between multiple compounds within a single plant. Here are some of the primary mechanisms:

Anti-inflammatory Effects

Many herbs exhibit anti-inflammatory properties by inhibiting pathways involved in the production of pro-inflammatory molecules like prostaglandins and cytokines. For example, curcumin from turmeric inhibits the NF-κB pathway, which plays a crucial role in inflammation.

Antioxidant Activity

Oxidative stress, caused by an imbalance between free radicals and antioxidants in the body, is implicated in many chronic diseases. Herbs rich in antioxidants, such as flavonoids and polyphenols, help neutralize free radicals and protect cells from damage. Green tea, rich in catechins, is a notable example.

Antimicrobial Properties

Herbs like garlic, thyme, and oregano contain compounds with antimicrobial properties that can combat bacterial, viral, and fungal infections. Allicin, a compound in garlic, has broad-spectrum antimicrobial activity.

Modulation of the Immune System

Certain herbs can modulate the immune system, enhancing its ability to fight infections and maintain homeostasis. Echinacea, for instance, stimulates the production of white blood cells and enhances immune response.

Hormonal Effects

Some herbs influence hormonal pathways, providing therapeutic benefits for conditions like menopause, menstrual disorders, and hormonal imbalances. Phytoestrogens in soy and red clover mimic estrogen and can alleviate menopausal symptoms.

Neuroprotective and Cognitive Effects

Herbs like ginkgo biloba and bacopa monnieri are known for their neuroprotective properties, improving cognitive function and protecting against neurodegenerative diseases. These effects are often mediated by enhanced blood flow, antioxidant activity, and modulation of neurotransmitter systems.

Evidence-Based Benefits

Scientific research has increasingly validated the health benefits of various herbs, leading to their integration into evidence-based medicine. Clinical trials and epidemiological studies provide robust data supporting the use of herbal remedies for various conditions.

Cardiovascular Health

Hawthorn, garlic, and green tea are examples of herbs with cardioprotective effects. They can lower blood pressure, reduce cholesterol levels, and improve blood vessel function.

Digestive Health

Herbs like ginger, peppermint, and fennel are effective in treating gastrointestinal issues such as nausea, bloating, and indigestion. Ginger, in particular, has well-documented anti-nausea effects, especially during pregnancy and chemotherapy.

Mental Health

Herbs like St. John's wort and valerian root are commonly used to manage depression and anxiety. St. John's wort has been shown to be as effective as conventional antidepressants for mild to moderate depression, with fewer side effects.

Immune Support

Echinacea and elderberry are popular herbs for boosting immune function and preventing infections. Studies have shown that elderberry can reduce the duration and severity of cold and flu symptoms.

Integrating Tradition and Science

The ongoing collaboration between traditional herbal medicine and modern scientific research is crucial for maximizing the therapeutic potential of herbs. Rigorous studies, including randomized controlled trials and systematic reviews, help establish the safety, efficacy, and optimal usage of herbal remedies. This integrative approach ensures that the ancient wisdom of herbal medicine continues to benefit contemporary health practices, offering natural solutions for a wide array of health challenges.

In conclusion, the science behind herbal remedies is a testament to the remarkable healing power of plants. By understanding the active compounds, mechanisms of action, and evidence-based benefits of herbs, we can harness their full potential to enhance our health and well-being. This knowledge bridges the gap between ancient traditions and modern science, paving the way for a holistic approach to medicine that honors the wisdom of nature.

Integrating Herbal Medicine into Modern Healthcare

As healthcare systems around the world grapple with the rising costs and side effects of conventional treatments, there is a growing interest in integrating herbal medicine into modern healthcare. Herbal remedies offer a complementary approach that can enhance the effectiveness of conventional treatments, reduce side effects, and provide holistic benefits. This chapter explores the ways in which herbal medicine can be effectively and safely incorporated into contemporary healthcare practices.

The Rationale for Integration

Addressing Chronic Diseases

Chronic diseases such as diabetes, heart disease, and arthritis are among the leading causes of morbidity and mortality worldwide. Herbal medicine offers promising solutions for managing these conditions. For instance, herbs like turmeric and ginger have potent anti-inflammatory properties that can help manage arthritis, while fenugreek and cinnamon can assist in blood sugar regulation for diabetes patients.

Reducing Side Effects

Many conventional medications come with a range of side effects that can significantly impact patients' quality of life. Herbal remedies, often with fewer side effects, can be used to mitigate these issues. For example, milk thistle is commonly used to protect the liver from damage caused by medications.

Enhancing Patient Compliance

Herbal medicines are often perceived as more natural and less invasive than synthetic drugs, which can enhance patient compliance. The use of herbs can also be tailored to individual preferences and cultural practices, making treatments more acceptable and accessible.

Integrative Approaches in Healthcare Settings

Collaborative Practices

Integrating herbal medicine into modern healthcare requires collaboration between conventional healthcare providers and herbal practitioners. This interdisciplinary approach ensures that patients receive comprehensive care. For example, an oncologist might work with an herbalist to develop a supportive treatment plan for a cancer patient experiencing side effects from chemotherapy.

Education and Training

Healthcare professionals need adequate training in herbal medicine to understand its benefits, limitations, and potential interactions with conventional drugs. Medical and nursing schools are beginning to incorporate courses on integrative medicine, including the use of herbs, into their curricula. Continuing education programs for practicing healthcare providers can also facilitate this knowledge integration.

Evidence-Based Practice

The integration of herbal medicine should be grounded in evidence-based practice. This involves rigorous scientific research to validate the efficacy and safety of herbal remedies. Healthcare providers should rely on high-quality studies, clinical trials, and meta-analyses to inform their use of herbs in treatment plans.

Practical Considerations

Safety and Quality Control

Ensuring the safety and quality of herbal products is paramount. Standardization of herbal extracts, rigorous testing for contaminants, and adherence to good manufacturing practices (GMP) are essential. Healthcare providers should recommend products from reputable sources and educate patients about the importance of quality control.

Dosage and Administration

Accurate dosing is crucial for the effectiveness and safety of herbal remedies. Unlike pharmaceuticals, the concentration of active ingredients in herbs can vary widely. Standardized extracts can help ensure consistent dosing. Healthcare providers should also guide patients on proper administration methods, such as preparing teas, tinctures, or capsules.

Monitoring and Follow-Up

Regular monitoring and follow-up are essential when incorporating herbal medicine into treatment plans. Healthcare providers should track patients' responses to herbal remedies, monitor for potential side effects, and adjust dosages as needed. This ongoing evaluation helps ensure that treatments are both effective and safe.

Case Studies and Success Stories

Integrative Oncology

In integrative oncology, herbal medicine is used to complement conventional cancer treatments. Herbs such as astragalus and ginseng are employed to boost immunity and enhance patients' energy levels during chemotherapy. Clinical studies have shown that these herbs can improve patients' quality of life and reduce treatment-related fatigue.

Pain Management

Chronic pain is a common issue that often requires a multi-faceted approach. Herbal remedies such as willow bark (a natural source of salicin, similar to aspirin) and capsaicin (derived from chili peppers) are used alongside conventional pain medications. Patients report significant pain relief and a reduction in the need for high doses of pharmaceuticals.

Mental Health

Herbal medicine offers valuable tools for managing mental health conditions like anxiety and depression. St. John's wort has been extensively studied for its antidepressant effects, while valerian root is commonly used for anxiety and insomnia. These herbs provide alternatives or adjuncts to conventional psychotropic medications, often with fewer side effects.

Overcoming Challenges

Regulatory Hurdles

One of the major challenges in integrating herbal medicine is navigating the regulatory landscape. Herbal products are regulated differently across countries, with varying standards for safety, efficacy, and quality. Harmonizing these regulations and ensuring rigorous oversight can help facilitate the integration of herbal medicine into mainstream healthcare.

Cultural Acceptance

Cultural acceptance of herbal medicine varies widely. In some cultures, herbal remedies are deeply ingrained in traditional healthcare practices, while in others, there may be skepticism or a lack of awareness. Education and public awareness campaigns can help bridge these gaps, promoting a more inclusive approach to healthcare.

Insurance and Reimbursement

Insurance coverage for herbal treatments is limited in many regions. Expanding coverage to include integrative approaches can make herbal medicine more accessible and affordable. Demonstrating the cost-effectiveness of herbal treatments through robust research can support policy changes and insurance reforms.

Integrating herbal medicine into modern healthcare offers a promising path toward more holistic and patient-centered care. By combining the strengths of conventional medicine with the wisdom of herbal remedies, healthcare providers can offer more comprehensive and effective treatments. This integrative approach not only enhances patient outcomes but also promotes a deeper connection to natural healing processes. As research continues to validate the benefits of herbal medicine, its role in contemporary healthcare is poised to expand, providing patients with safe, effective, and holistic treatment options.

Introduction to Understanding Herbal Medicine

Herbal medicine, the art and science of using plants for their therapeutic properties, has been a cornerstone of healthcare for millennia. From ancient apothecaries to modern health food stores, herbs have provided remedies for a myriad of ailments and have played a vital role in maintaining health and well-being. In a world increasingly reliant on pharmaceuticals and advanced medical technologies, there is a growing recognition of the value of natural and holistic approaches to health. Understanding herbal medicine allows us to tap into this ancient wisdom, blending it with contemporary scientific insights to enhance our overall wellness.

This book is designed to demystify the complex world of herbal medicine, making it accessible and practical for everyone, whether you're a seasoned practitioner or a curious newcomer. We will explore the rich history of herbal medicine, from its roots in ancient civilizations to its resurgence in modern healthcare. By understanding the science behind how herbs work, you will gain a deeper appreciation of their healing potential and learn how to integrate them safely and effectively into your daily life.

Throughout these pages, we will delve into the diverse array of herbs used in traditional and contemporary practices, examining their active compounds, health benefits, and potential uses. You will discover how to identify, prepare, and use these botanical treasures, from common kitchen spices to exotic medicinal plants. By the end of this journey, you will have a comprehensive understanding of herbal medicine and the confidence to harness its power for your health and the well-being of your loved ones.

Join us as we embark on this enlightening journey into the world of herbal medicine. Together, we will unlock the secrets of nature's pharmacy and embrace a holistic approach to health that honors the wisdom of the past while embracing the advancements of the present. Welcome to a deeper understanding of the healing power of herbs.

How Herbs Work in the Body

Herbs have been used for centuries to heal and support health, but understanding how they work in the body reveals the intricate and fascinating ways in which plants interact with our biological systems. The therapeutic effects of herbs are rooted in their complex chemical compositions, which include a variety of active compounds. These compounds work synergistically to produce physiological changes, promote healing, and maintain balance within the body.

Active Compounds in Herbs

Alkaloids

Alkaloids are potent nitrogen-containing compounds that have significant physiological effects. They often act on the nervous system and can provide pain relief, stimulate or relax muscles, and influence mood and perception. For example, morphine, derived from the opium poppy, is a powerful analgesic, while caffeine from coffee and tea is a well-known stimulant.

Flavonoids

Flavonoids are a group of polyphenolic compounds that exhibit strong antioxidant properties. They protect cells from oxidative damage caused by free radicals, reduce inflammation, and support cardiovascular health. Quercetin, found in onions and apples, is a widely studied flavonoid known for its anti-inflammatory and antihistamine effects.

Terpenes and Terpenoids

These aromatic compounds contribute to the scent and flavor of herbs and have diverse therapeutic properties. Terpenes can act as anti-inflammatory, antiviral, and antibacterial agents. For example, menthol from peppermint oil provides a cooling sensation and pain relief, while cannabinoids from cannabis interact with the endocannabinoid system to regulate various physiological processes.

Glycosides

Glycosides are compounds that yield active substances upon hydrolysis. They include cardiac glycosides, like digoxin from foxglove, which are used to treat heart failure and arrhythmias by increasing the force of cardiac contractions. Saponins, another type of glycoside, have immune-boosting and cholesterol-lowering effects.

Tannins

Tannins are astringent compounds that can constrict tissues and reduce inflammation. They are commonly found in herbs like witch hazel and oak bark and are used to treat wounds, diarrhea, and skin conditions.

Mechanisms of Action

Anti-inflammatory Effects

Many herbs exert anti-inflammatory effects by inhibiting enzymes and signaling pathways involved in the production of pro-inflammatory molecules such as prostaglandins and cytokines. Turmeric's active compound, curcumin, for instance, inhibits the NF-κB pathway, a key regulator of inflammation.

Antioxidant Activity

Herbs rich in antioxidants neutralize free radicals, thereby preventing cellular damage and reducing the risk of chronic diseases. Antioxidants like vitamin C, vitamin E, and polyphenols from herbs scavenge free radicals, thereby protecting DNA, proteins, and lipids from oxidative stress.

Antimicrobial Properties

Certain herbs possess compounds with antimicrobial activity, capable of combating bacteria, viruses, fungi, and parasites. For example, allicin in garlic has been shown to have broad-spectrum antibacterial and antiviral properties, making it useful for infections and immune support.

Modulation of the Immune System

Herbs can modulate the immune system, enhancing its ability to fight infections and maintain homeostasis. Echinacea, for instance, is known to stimulate the production and activity of white blood cells, thereby boosting the immune response.

Hormonal Effects

Some herbs influence hormonal pathways, providing therapeutic benefits for conditions like menopause, menstrual disorders, and hormonal imbalances. Phytoestrogens in soy and red clover mimic estrogen, helping to alleviate symptoms of menopause.

Neuroprotective and Cognitive Effects

Herbs like ginkgo biloba and bacopa monnieri are renowned for their neuroprotective and cognitive-enhancing properties. They improve blood flow to the brain, reduce oxidative stress, and modulate neurotransmitter activity, supporting memory, focus, and overall cognitive function.

Synergy and the Whole Herb Concept

One of the unique aspects of herbal medicine is the concept of synergy, where the combined effect of all the compounds in an herb is greater than the sum of their individual effects. This holistic approach considers the whole plant and its various constituents working together to produce balanced and effective therapeutic outcomes. This is in contrast to the reductionist approach of isolating single active compounds, as seen in conventional pharmaceuticals.

Practical Application and Safety

Understanding how herbs work in the body is crucial for their effective and safe use. Dosage, preparation methods, and potential interactions with medications need careful consideration. While herbs are generally safe, they can have potent effects and interact with other treatments. Consulting with healthcare providers and qualified herbalists ensures that herbs are used appropriately and effectively.

Herbs work in the body through a complex interplay of active compounds that influence various physiological processes. Their anti-inflammatory, antioxidant, antimicrobial, immune-modulating, hormonal, and neuroprotective properties demonstrate the vast potential of herbal medicine. By harnessing these natural remedies, we can support our health in a holistic and balanced manner, drawing on the wisdom of traditional practices and the insights of modern science.

Preparing Herbal Remedies: Teas, Tinctures, Salves, and More

The art of preparing herbal remedies is a time-honored tradition that allows us to harness the healing properties of plants in various forms. Whether you're brewing a soothing tea, crafting a potent tincture, or creating a healing salve, understanding the methods of preparation is essential for unlocking the therapeutic potential of herbs. This chapter explores the different techniques for preparing herbal remedies, offering practical guidance and tips for each method.

Herbal Teas

Overview

Herbal teas, also known as infusions or tisanes, are one of the simplest and most effective ways to enjoy the benefits of herbs. They are made by steeping herbs in hot water, allowing their active compounds to be extracted into the liquid.

Preparation

1. Choosing Herbs: Select fresh or dried herbs. Common choices include chamomile for relaxation, peppermint for digestion, and ginger for anti-inflammatory benefits.

2. Measurement: Use about 1-2 teaspoons of dried herbs or 1-2 tablespoons of fresh herbs per cup

of water.

3. Steeping: Place the herbs in a teapot or infuser. Pour boiling water over them and cover. Let steep for 5-15 minutes, depending on the herb and desired strength.

4. Straining: Strain the herbs using a fine mesh strainer or remove the infuser. Sweeten with honey or lemon if desired.

Tips

- For roots and bark, such as ginger or cinnamon, simmer the herbs in water for 10-20 minutes instead of steeping.
- Store dried herbs in a cool, dark place to preserve their potency.

Tinctures

Overview

Tinctures are concentrated liquid extracts made by soaking herbs in alcohol or glycerin. They are potent, shelf-stable, and easy to use, making them a popular choice for herbal remedies.

Preparation

1. Choosing Herbs and Solvent: Use dried or fresh herbs. High-proof alcohol (like vodka or brandy) is commonly used, but glycerin can be an alternative for alcohol-free tinctures.

2. Measurement: Fill a glass jar about 1/3 to 1/2 full with chopped fresh herbs or 1/4 full with dried herbs. Fill the jar with alcohol or glycerin, ensuring the herbs are fully submerged.

3. Infusing: Seal the jar tightly and place it in a cool, dark place. Shake the jar daily to help with extraction. Let it infuse for 4-6 weeks.

4. Straining: Strain the mixture through a cheesecloth or fine mesh strainer, pressing the herbs to extract as much liquid as possible. Transfer the tincture to a dark glass bottle for storage.

Tips

- Label your tinctures with the herb name and date of preparation.
- A typical dosage is 1-2 droppers full (about 1/4 to 1/2 teaspoon) diluted in water or juice.

Salves

Overview

Herbal salves are topical preparations made by infusing herbs into oils and combining them with beeswax to create a soothing, healing ointment. They are excellent for skin conditions, wounds, and muscle pain.

Preparation

1. Choosing Herbs and Oils: Select herbs with desired properties (e.g., calendula for healing, arnica for pain relief) and a carrier oil (such as olive, coconut, or jojoba oil).

2. Infusing the Oil:
- Slow Method: Fill a jar with herbs and cover with oil. Let it infuse in a sunny windowsill for 4-6 weeks, shaking occasionally.
- Quick Method: Gently heat the herbs and oil in a double boiler for 2-4 hours, keeping the temperature below 140°F to avoid damaging the herbs.

3. Straining: Strain the oil through a cheesecloth or fine mesh strainer to remove the herbs.

4. Making the Salve:
- Heat the infused oil in a double boiler and add beeswax (approximately 1 ounce of beeswax per 4 ounces of oil).
- Stir until the beeswax is fully melted and blended.
- Pour the mixture into tins or jars and let it cool and solidify.

Tips

- For added benefits, you can mix essential oils into the salve before it cools.
- Store salves in a cool, dark place to extend their shelf life.

Other Herbal Preparations

Syrups

Herbal syrups are sweet, concentrated extracts often used to soothe coughs and sore throats.

Preparation:
1. Make a strong herbal decoction by simmering herbs in water.
2. Strain the liquid and return it to the heat.
3. Add honey or sugar (at a 1:1 ratio to the liquid) and simmer until dissolved and thickened.
4. Store in a sterilized bottle in the refrigerator.

Poultices and Compresses

Poultices and compresses involve applying herbs directly to the skin to reduce inflammation, draw out infections, or promote healing.

Preparation:
1. Poultice: Mash fresh herbs or mix dried herbs with hot water to form a paste. Apply directly to the skin and cover with a clean cloth.
2. Compress: Soak a cloth in a strong herbal infusion or decoction and apply it to the affected area.

Capsules

Capsules are a convenient way to consume powdered herbs, particularly those with a strong taste or when precise dosing is needed.

Preparation:
1. Fill empty gelatin or vegetarian capsules with powdered herbs using a capsule machine.
2. Store in a cool, dry place.

Preparing herbal remedies is a rewarding and practical way to incorporate the healing power of plants into your daily life. Whether you are crafting a comforting tea, a potent tincture, or a soothing salve, understanding the methods and techniques involved ensures that you can create effective and safe herbal preparations. With a little practice and knowledge, you can harness the benefits of herbs and take an active role in your health and well-being.

Safety and Dosage Considerations

The use of herbal remedies offers a natural and holistic approach to health, but it is essential to approach their use with an understanding of safety and proper dosage. While herbs can provide significant therapeutic benefits, they also contain potent bioactive compounds that can cause adverse effects if not used correctly. This chapter outlines key safety considerations and guidelines for determining appropriate dosages to ensure that herbal remedies are used effectively and safely.

General Safety Guidelines

Quality and Source

1. Reputable Suppliers: Purchase herbs from reputable suppliers who follow good manufacturing practices (GMP). This ensures that the products are free from contaminants such as heavy metals, pesticides, and adulterants.
2. Organic and Wildcrafted: Choose organic or wildcrafted herbs whenever possible to avoid exposure to harmful chemicals.
3. Proper Identification: Ensure that the herbs are correctly identified, as misidentification can lead to the use of toxic plants.

Allergies and Sensitivities

1. Allergy Testing: If you have a history of allergies, perform a patch test before using a new herb topically. Apply a small amount of the herb preparation to the skin and wait 24 hours to check for any reaction.
2. Food Sensitivities: Be aware of any food sensitivities, as some herbs can cause reactions similar to those of foods you are allergic to.

Interaction with Medications

1. Consult Healthcare Providers: Always consult with a healthcare provider or a qualified herbalist before combining herbal remedies with prescription medications. Some herbs can interact with medications, altering their effects or causing side effects.
2. Herb-Drug Interactions: Be aware of common herb-drug interactions. For example, St. John's wort can decrease the effectiveness of oral contraceptives and certain antidepressants, while ginkgo biloba can increase the risk of bleeding when taken with blood thinners.

Special Populations

1. Pregnancy and Breastfeeding: Certain herbs are contraindicated during pregnancy and breastfeeding due to potential risks to the mother and child. Always consult with a healthcare provider before using herbs in these situations.
2. Children and Elderly: Dosages for children and the elderly may need to be adjusted due to differences in metabolism and sensitivity. Use herbs with caution and under professional guidance in these age groups.

Determining Dosage

Factors Influencing Dosage

1. Age, Weight, and Health Status: Consider the individual's age, weight, and overall health when determining the appropriate dosage. Children, elderly individuals, and those with chronic health conditions may require lower dosages.
2. Herb Potency: The potency of the herb, which can vary based on its form (fresh, dried, extract) and preparation method, influences the appropriate dosage.
3. Therapeutic Goal: The therapeutic goal (e.g., acute symptom relief vs. long-term maintenance) will also determine the appropriate dosage and duration of use.

General Dosage Guidelines

1. Teas and Infusions: Use 1-2 teaspoons of dried herbs or 1-2 tablespoons of fresh herbs per cup of water. Drink 1-3 cups per day, depending on the herb and the condition being treated.
2. Tinctures: A typical dosage is 1-2 droppers full (approximately 1/4 to 1/2 teaspoon) diluted in water or juice, taken 2-3 times per day.
3. Capsules: Follow the dosage recommendations provided by the manufacturer. Common dosages range from 500 mg to 2000 mg per day, depending on the herb.
4. Salves and Topicals: Apply a small amount to the affected area 2-3 times per day, adjusting based on skin sensitivity and response.

Adjusting Dosage

1. Start Low, Go Slow: Begin with a lower dosage to gauge the body's response, especially when using a new herb. Gradually increase the dosage if needed and if no adverse effects occur.
2. Monitor for Side Effects: Keep track of any side effects or adverse reactions. If any occur, reduce the dosage or discontinue use and consult a healthcare provider.
3. Duration of Use: Some herbs are suitable for long-term use, while others should only be used short-term. Follow recommendations for the duration of use based on the herb and the condition being treated.

Recognizing Adverse Reactions

1. Common Side Effects: Mild digestive upset, headaches, or skin reactions can occur when using herbs. Monitor for these and adjust dosage as needed.
2. Serious Reactions: Rare but serious reactions can include allergic reactions (e.g., hives, difficulty breathing), liver toxicity, or severe gastrointestinal issues. Discontinue use immediately and seek medical attention if any of these occur.

The safe and effective use of herbal remedies requires careful consideration of quality, potential interactions, appropriate dosages, and individual health needs. By following these guidelines and consulting with healthcare professionals when necessary, you can enjoy the therapeutic benefits of herbs while minimizing the risks. With knowledge and mindfulness, herbal medicine can be a powerful tool for supporting health and well-being.

Sourcing Quality Herbs: Wildcrafting and Ethical Harvesting

The quality of herbs used in herbal remedies directly impacts their efficacy and safety. While purchasing from reputable suppliers is common, another option is to wildcraft or ethically harvest herbs directly from their natural habitats. Wildcrafting involves gathering plants from their native environments, while ethical harvesting emphasizes sustainable practices that protect both the plant populations and the surrounding ecosystems. This chapter explores the principles of wildcrafting and ethical harvesting, offering guidance on how to responsibly source high-quality herbs for your herbal preparations.

Understanding Wildcrafting and Ethical Harvesting

Wildcrafting

1. Definition: Wildcrafting, also known as foraging, involves gathering medicinal plants from their natural habitats, such as forests, meadows, and mountains.
2. Connection to Nature: Wildcrafting fosters a deep connection to nature and the land, allowing herbalists to develop a deeper understanding of plant ecosystems and their medicinal properties.
3. Challenges: Wildcrafting requires knowledge of plant identification, ethical considerations, and sustainable harvesting practices to ensure the long-term health of plant populations.

Ethical Harvesting

1. Sustainability: Ethical harvesting emphasizes sustainable practices that minimize the impact on plant populations and their habitats.
2. Respect for Nature: It involves respecting the natural lifecycle of plants, harvesting only what is needed, and leaving enough plants to ensure their survival and reproduction.
3. Cultural and Indigenous Perspectives: Many indigenous cultures have traditional knowledge and practices for ethically harvesting medicinal plants, passed down through generations.

Principles of Ethical Harvesting

Plant Identification

1. Botanical Knowledge: Develop a thorough understanding of plant identification, including key botanical features, habitat preferences, and seasonal variations.
2. Field Guides and Resources: Use reputable field guides, plant identification apps, and online resources to aid in identification and verification.

Sustainable Harvesting Practices

1. Selective Harvesting: Harvest plants selectively, taking only what is needed and leaving enough to ensure their continued growth and reproduction.
2. Avoid Overharvesting: Be mindful of the vulnerability of plant populations and avoid overharvesting in sensitive areas or for rare or endangered species.
3. Harvesting Ethics: Follow ethical guidelines such as the "leave no trace" principle, minimizing disturbance to the ecosystem and respecting the rights of indigenous communities.

Seasonal Considerations

1. Timing: Harvest plants at the appropriate time of year, when they are at their peak potency and abundance.
2. Life Cycle: Understand the lifecycle of the plant, including when it flowers, fruits, and goes dormant, to ensure sustainable harvesting practices.

Location and Habitat

1. Responsible Access: Obtain permission from landowners or land management agencies before

wildcrafting on private or protected lands.
2. Habitat Preservation: Choose harvesting sites carefully, avoiding areas with pollution, heavy foot traffic, or other disturbances that could harm plant populations or the ecosystem.

Best Practices for Ethical Harvesting

Research and Education

1. Local Regulations: Familiarize yourself with local regulations and guidelines for wildcrafting and harvesting medicinal plants.
2. Training and Mentorship: Seek out training programs, workshops, or mentorship opportunities with experienced herbalists or indigenous elders to learn ethical harvesting practices.

Sustainable Harvesting Techniques

1. Hand Harvesting: Use hand tools or scissors to carefully harvest plants, minimizing damage to roots, stems, and surrounding vegetation.
2. Seed Saving: Collect and propagate seeds to support plant regeneration and biodiversity in your local ecosystem.

Documentation and Record-Keeping

1. Harvesting Logs: Keep detailed records of harvested plants, including location, date, quantity, and any observations about the habitat and plant populations.
2. Ethical Code of Conduct: Develop a personal or community code of conduct for ethical harvesting practices, emphasizing stewardship, respect, and reciprocity.

Sourcing quality herbs through wildcrafting and ethical harvesting offers a deeply rewarding connection to nature and the healing power of plants. By adhering to principles of sustainability, respect, and stewardship, herbalists can ensure the long-term viability of plant populations and protect the delicate balance of ecosystems. Through education, training, and a commitment to ethical practices, we can cultivate a harmonious relationship with the natural world and continue to benefit from its abundant medicinal treasures for generations to come.

Introduction to Herbal Remedies for Common Ailments

In a world where modern medicine often takes center stage, the wisdom of traditional herbal remedies continues to offer profound insights into the healing potential of nature. Herbal remedies have been used for centuries to address a wide range of common ailments, providing gentle yet effective relief for everything from minor discomforts to chronic conditions. In this comprehensive guide, we delve into the world of herbal medicine, exploring the diverse array of plants and remedies that can support health and well-being.

Embracing Nature's Pharmacy

Herbs have long been revered for their ability to heal, nourish, and restore balance within the body. From the soothing properties of chamomile to the immune-boosting effects of echinacea, each plant offers a unique blend of therapeutic compounds that can address specific health concerns. By tapping into nature's pharmacy, we gain access to a wealth of botanical treasures that can complement and enhance our overall health.

A Holistic Approach to Wellness

Herbal remedies offer more than just symptom relief; they provide a holistic approach to wellness that considers the interconnectedness of the body, mind, and spirit. By addressing the root causes of illness and supporting the body's innate healing mechanisms, herbs empower us to take an active role in our health journey. Whether used alone or in conjunction with conventional treatments, herbal remedies offer a gentle and natural alternative for promoting vitality and resilience.

Navigating the World of Herbal Medicine

While the abundance of herbal remedies may seem overwhelming at first, this guide aims to demystify the process of selecting, preparing, and using herbs for common ailments. From herbal teas and tinctures to salves and syrups, we explore a variety of preparations and techniques that allow you to harness the healing power of plants in your own home. With a focus on safety, efficacy, and sustainability, we provide practical guidance for incorporating herbal remedies into your daily wellness routine.

Empowering Self-Care

At its core, herbal medicine is about empowerment – empowering individuals to take control of their health and well-being through natural, accessible, and sustainable means. Whether you're seeking relief from a nagging cough, soothing support for digestive discomfort, or immune-boosting tonics to ward off illness, this guide equips you with the knowledge and tools to address common ailments with confidence and ease.

The Journey Ahead

Join us on a journey through the enchanting world of herbal remedies, where ancient wisdom meets modern science in a harmonious dance of healing and renewal. Together, let us rediscover the transformative power of nature's botanical bounty and embark on a path toward greater vitality, resilience, and well-being. Welcome to Herbal Remedies for Common Ailments – your trusted companion on the path to natural health and vitality.

Herbal Remedies for Allergies and Respiratory Issues

Allergies and respiratory issues are common ailments that can significantly impact quality of life, from seasonal allergies causing sneezing and congestion to chronic respiratory conditions like asthma and bronchitis. While conventional treatments provide relief for many, herbal remedies offer a natural and holistic approach to supporting respiratory health and alleviating allergy symptoms. In this chapter, we explore a variety of herbs and herbal preparations that can help soothe inflammation, clear congestion, and strengthen the respiratory system.

Understanding Allergies and Respiratory Issues

Allergies

1. Seasonal Allergies: Seasonal allergies, also known as hay fever or allergic rhinitis, occur when the immune system overreacts to airborne allergens such as pollen, mold, or pet dander.
2. Symptoms: Common symptoms include sneezing, runny or stuffy nose, itchy eyes, and coughing.

Respiratory Issues

1. Asthma: Asthma is a chronic condition characterized by inflammation and narrowing of the

airways, leading to difficulty breathing, wheezing, and chest tightness.
2. Bronchitis: Bronchitis is an inflammation of the bronchial tubes, often caused by viral or bacterial infections, resulting in coughing, chest discomfort, and mucus production.

Herbal Remedies for Allergies and Respiratory Health

Nettle (Urtica dioica)

- Properties: Nettle is a natural antihistamine and anti-inflammatory herb, making it effective for relieving allergy symptoms such as sneezing and itching.
- Preparation: Drink nettle tea or take nettle supplements to reduce allergic reactions and promote respiratory health.

Licorice Root (Glycyrrhiza glabra)

- Properties: Licorice root has expectorant and anti-inflammatory properties, making it useful for soothing coughs and reducing inflammation in the respiratory tract.
- Preparation: Drink licorice root tea or take licorice root supplements to relieve coughs and promote respiratory comfort.

Elderberry (Sambucus nigra)

- Properties: Elderberry is rich in antioxidants and has immune-boosting properties, making it beneficial for preventing and treating respiratory infections.
- Preparation: Take elderberry syrup or supplements to support immune function and reduce the severity and duration of respiratory illnesses.

Eucalyptus (Eucalyptus globulus)

- Properties: Eucalyptus has decongestant and expectorant properties, making it effective for clearing nasal congestion and relieving coughs.
- Preparation: Inhale eucalyptus essential oil vapors or use eucalyptus chest rubs to ease respiratory discomfort and promote clearer breathing.

Peppermint (Mentha piperita)

- Properties: Peppermint has antispasmodic and decongestant properties, making it helpful for relieving coughs, sinus congestion, and breathing difficulties.
- Preparation: Drink peppermint tea or inhale peppermint essential oil vapors to soothe respiratory symptoms and promote relaxation.

Herbal Preparations and Usage Tips

- Teas: Steep herbs in hot water to make soothing teas that can be enjoyed throughout the day.
- Tinctures: Take herbal tinctures diluted in water or juice for a concentrated dose of therapeutic benefits.
- Steam Inhalation: Add herbs to hot water and inhale the steam to relieve congestion and promote respiratory comfort.
- Topical Applications: Use herbal chest rubs or balms to soothe chest congestion and ease breathing discomfort.

Safety Considerations

- Dosage: Follow recommended dosage guidelines for each herb to avoid adverse effects.
- Allergies: Be aware of potential allergies or sensitivities to specific herbs and discontinue use if any adverse reactions occur.
- Interactions: Consult with a healthcare provider before using herbal remedies, especially if you are pregnant, nursing, or taking medications.

Herbal remedies offer valuable support for allergies and respiratory issues, providing natural alternatives to conventional treatments. By incorporating herbs into your daily routine, you can soothe inflammation, clear congestion, and strengthen your respiratory system, promoting greater comfort and well-being. With a holistic approach to respiratory health that addresses both symptoms and underlying imbalances, herbal medicine offers a gentle and effective solution for common respiratory ailments.

Nettles: Nature's Allergy Reliever

Introduction

Nettles, with their humble appearance and often-overlooked presence, hold within their vibrant green leaves a potent remedy for allergies and a plethora of other health benefits. Despite their stinging reputation, nettles (scientifically known as Urtica dioica) have been revered for centuries as a medicinal herb, celebrated for their ability to alleviate symptoms of seasonal allergies, support urinary health, and provide a rich source of nutrients. In this chapter, we uncover the remarkable healing properties of nettles and explore how this unassuming plant can offer relief and vitality to those who seek it.

Understanding Nettles

Botanical Background: Nettles belong to the genus Urtica and are found in temperate regions around the world. They typically grow in nitrogen-rich soil and are characterized by their serrated leaves and tiny, stinging hairs that release histamine upon contact with the skin.

Medicinal Properties: Despite their sting, nettles are prized for their medicinal properties. Rich in vitamins (including A, C, and K), minerals (such as iron, calcium, and magnesium), and flavonoids, nettles possess anti-inflammatory, antihistamine, and diuretic properties that make them invaluable in herbal medicine.

Harnessing the Power of Nettles

Allergy Relief: Nettles are perhaps best known for their ability to relieve symptoms of seasonal allergies, including sneezing, itching, and congestion. Studies suggest that nettles may inhibit the release of histamine and other inflammatory compounds, offering natural relief without the side effects associated with conventional antihistamines.

Urinary Support: Nettles have a long history of use in supporting urinary health. As a gentle diuretic, nettles help to flush toxins from the body, making them useful for conditions such as urinary tract infections and kidney stones.

Nutritional Support: Nettles are a nutritional powerhouse, providing essential vitamins and minerals that support overall health and vitality. Whether consumed as a tea, added to soups and stews, or taken as a supplement, nettles offer a convenient way to boost nutrient intake and support optimal wellness.

How to Use Nettles

Nettle Tea: Steep dried nettle leaves in hot water to make a soothing tea that can be enjoyed daily. Nettle tea is a refreshing and nourishing beverage that can be enjoyed on its own or combined with other herbs for added benefits.

Nettle Supplements: Nettle supplements, available in capsule or tincture form, offer a convenient way to incorporate nettles into your daily routine. Follow recommended dosage guidelines to ensure safe and effective use.

Nettle Infusions: For a more potent remedy, consider making a nettle infusion by steeping a larger quantity of nettles in hot water for an extended period. This concentrated herbal preparation can be used as a tonic to support overall health and well-being.

Safety Considerations

While nettles are generally safe for most people, it is essential to exercise caution when handling fresh nettles due to their stinging hairs. If harvesting nettles yourself, wear gloves and long sleeves to avoid skin irritation. Additionally, individuals with certain medical conditions or those taking medications should consult with a healthcare professional before using nettles as a supplement.

Nettles, with their remarkable healing properties and versatile uses, offer a natural solution for allergies, urinary health, and overall well-being. Whether enjoyed as a nourishing tea, incorporated into culinary creations, or taken as a supplement, nettles provide a gentle and effective remedy that honors the wisdom of nature. By embracing the power of nettles, we can tap into a rich source of vitality and resilience, supporting our health and thriving in harmony with the natural world.

Butterbur: Nature's Migraine Soother

Introduction

Butterbur, with its broad leaves and cheerful clusters of flowers, is not only a picturesque addition to the landscape but also a powerful ally in the fight against migraines and other ailments. This remarkable herb, scientifically known as Petasites hybridus, has been used for centuries in traditional medicine to alleviate headaches, reduce inflammation, and support respiratory health. In this chapter, we explore the therapeutic properties of butterbur and its potential to offer relief and comfort to those who suffer from migraines and other conditions.

Understanding Butterbur

Botanical Background: Butterbur is a perennial herb native to Europe, Asia, and parts of North America. It belongs to the Asteraceae family and is characterized by its large, heart-shaped leaves and pink or white flowers. The name "butterbur" is thought to stem from its traditional use in wrapping butter to keep it cool during warmer months.

Medicinal Properties: Butterbur contains bioactive compounds, including petasin and isopetasin, which possess anti-inflammatory and antispasmodic properties. These compounds are believed to help relax blood vessels, reduce muscle spasms, and inhibit the release of inflammatory substances, making butterbur particularly effective for relieving migraine headaches.

Harnessing the Power of Butterbur

Migraine Relief: Butterbur has gained recognition for its ability to reduce the frequency, severity, and duration of migraines. Studies have shown that butterbur extract can be as effective as conventional migraine medications, with fewer side effects. By inhibiting the constriction of blood vessels and reducing inflammation in the brain, butterbur offers natural relief for migraine sufferers.

Respiratory Support: Butterbur has also been used traditionally to support respiratory health and alleviate symptoms of asthma and allergies. Its anti-inflammatory properties help to reduce airway inflammation and bronchial spasms, making it beneficial for conditions such as asthma, bronchitis, and allergic rhinitis.

Urinary Health: In addition to its effects on migraines and respiratory issues, butterbur may also support urinary health. As a diuretic, butterbur helps to increase urine flow and flush toxins from the body, making it useful for conditions such as urinary tract infections and kidney stones.

How to Use Butterbur

Butterbur Extract: Butterbur extract, standardized to contain specific concentrations of petasin and isopetasin, is available in capsule or tablet form. Follow recommended dosage guidelines to ensure safe and effective use. Look for products that are labeled "PA-free," as some butterbur supplements may contain pyrrolizidine alkaloids (PAs), which can be toxic to the liver.

Butterbur Tea: While less common, butterbur tea can be made by steeping dried butterbur leaves in hot water. However, due to the presence of PAs, it is essential to use caution and ensure that the tea is made from a reputable source.

Safety Considerations

While butterbur is generally considered safe when used appropriately, it is crucial to choose products that are PA-free to avoid potential liver toxicity. Pregnant and breastfeeding women should avoid using butterbur due to a lack of safety data. Additionally, individuals with certain medical conditions or those taking medications should consult with a healthcare professional before using butterbur supplements.

Butterbur, with its remarkable ability to soothe migraines, support respiratory health, and promote urinary wellness, offers a natural solution for a variety of ailments. Whether taken as a supplement or used in traditional herbal preparations, butterbur harnesses the power of nature to provide relief and comfort to those who seek it. By embracing the healing potential of butterbur, we can find respite from pain, support our overall well-being, and thrive in harmony with the natural world.

Mullein: Nature's Respiratory Healer

Introduction

Mullein, with its tall stalks and soft, fuzzy leaves, stands as a sentinel of healing in the world of herbal medicine. This versatile herb, scientifically known as Verbascum thapsus, has been revered for centuries for its ability to support respiratory health, soothe inflammation, and provide relief from various ailments. In this chapter, we delve into the remarkable properties of mullein and explore how this humble plant can offer comfort and healing to those in need.

Understanding Mullein

Botanical Background: Mullein is a biennial plant native to Europe, Asia, and North Africa but has since naturalized in many parts of the world. It belongs to the Scrophulariaceae family and is characterized by its tall flower spikes, velvety leaves, and cheerful yellow flowers. Mullein has a long history of use in traditional medicine, with records dating back to ancient civilizations such as the Greeks and Romans.

Medicinal Properties: Mullein contains a variety of bioactive compounds, including saponins, flavonoids, and mucilage, which contribute to its therapeutic effects. These compounds have expectorant, demulcent, and anti-inflammatory properties, making mullein particularly beneficial for respiratory conditions such as coughs, bronchitis, and asthma.

Harnessing the Power of Mullein

Respiratory Support: Mullein is perhaps best known for its ability to support respiratory health and alleviate symptoms of respiratory conditions. Its expectorant properties help to loosen and expel mucus from the lungs, making it useful for coughs, chest congestion, and bronchial infections. Mullein also has anti-inflammatory effects, which can help to soothe irritated airways and reduce coughing.

Ear Health: In addition to its respiratory benefits, mullein has traditionally been used to support ear health. Mullein oil, made by infusing mullein flowers in olive or almond oil, can be used topically to soothe earaches and reduce inflammation in the ear canal. Its mild analgesic and antimicrobial properties make it a gentle and effective remedy for ear discomfort.

Skin Care: Mullein has also been used topically to support skin health and promote wound healing. Mullein poultices or compresses can be applied to minor wounds, burns, or insect bites to reduce inflammation and promote tissue repair. The mucilage found in mullein leaves helps to hydrate and protect the skin, making it beneficial for dry, irritated skin conditions.

How to Use Mullein

Mullein Tea: Mullein tea can be made by steeping dried mullein leaves or flowers in hot water for 10-15 minutes. This soothing herbal infusion can be enjoyed up to three times per day to support respiratory health and alleviate coughs and congestion.

Mullein Tincture: Mullein tincture, made by extracting mullein leaves or flowers in alcohol or glycerin, offers a concentrated dose of mullein's therapeutic compounds. Take mullein tincture diluted in water or juice, following recommended dosage guidelines.

Mullein Oil: Mullein oil can be made by infusing dried mullein flowers in a carrier oil such as olive or almond oil. Apply mullein oil topically to the chest for respiratory support or to the ears for earaches and inflammation.

Safety Considerations

Mullein is generally considered safe when used appropriately, but individuals with certain medical conditions or those taking medications should consult with a healthcare professional before using mullein supplements. Pregnant or breastfeeding women should also exercise caution when using mullein. Additionally, avoid harvesting mullein from contaminated or polluted areas, as the plant may absorb toxins from the soil.

Mullein, with its gentle yet potent healing properties, offers a natural solution for respiratory ailments, earaches, and skin conditions. Whether enjoyed as a soothing tea, applied topically as an oil, or taken as a tincture, mullein provides comfort and relief to those seeking healing from nature's pharmacy. By embracing the power of mullein, we can support our respiratory health, soothe our bodies, and reconnect with the wisdom of the natural world.

Eucalyptus: Nature's Respiratory Revitalizer

Introduction

Eucalyptus, with its distinctive scent and cooling properties, stands tall as a symbol of vitality and rejuvenation in the world of herbal medicine. This versatile tree, belonging to the genus Eucalyptus and native to Australia, has been revered for centuries for its ability to support respiratory health, ease congestion, and promote overall well-being. In this chapter, we explore the remarkable properties of eucalyptus and how this aromatic herb can offer comfort and relief to those seeking natural respiratory support.

Understanding Eucalyptus

Botanical Background: Eucalyptus is a diverse genus comprising over 700 species of evergreen trees and shrubs, many of which are valued for their medicinal properties. The most commonly used species for therapeutic purposes include Eucalyptus globulus, Eucalyptus radiata, and Eucalyptus smithii. Eucalyptus trees are characterized by their smooth bark, aromatic leaves, and small, white flowers.

Medicinal Properties: Eucalyptus leaves contain a high concentration of essential oils, including eucalyptol (also known as cineole), which gives the plant its distinctive scent and therapeutic properties. Eucalyptus oil has antimicrobial, expectorant, and decongestant properties, making it highly effective for respiratory conditions such as coughs, colds, and sinus congestion.

Harnessing the Power of Eucalyptus

Respiratory Support: Eucalyptus is renowned for its ability to support respiratory health and alleviate symptoms of respiratory conditions. Inhalation of eucalyptus oil vapors helps to open up the airways, reduce inflammation, and promote clearer breathing. Eucalyptus is particularly beneficial for coughs, chest congestion, sinusitis, and bronchitis.

Immune Boosting: Eucalyptus oil has antimicrobial properties that help to combat bacteria, viruses, and fungi. By supporting the body's immune response, eucalyptus can help to prevent and shorten the duration of respiratory infections, including the common cold and flu.

Mental Clarity and Focus: The invigorating aroma of eucalyptus has a stimulating effect on the mind, promoting mental clarity, focus, and alertness. Inhalation of eucalyptus oil can help to combat fatigue, improve concentration, and enhance cognitive function.

How to Use Eucalyptus

Eucalyptus Inhalation: Add a few drops of eucalyptus essential oil to a bowl of hot water and inhale the steam to relieve congestion and promote clearer breathing. Alternatively, add eucalyptus oil to a diffuser to enjoy the benefits of aromatherapy throughout the day.

Eucalyptus Chest Rub: Mix eucalyptus essential oil with a carrier oil such as coconut or almond oil and apply the mixture to the chest and throat to soothe congestion and coughing. This natural chest rub can provide relief from respiratory discomfort and promote relaxation.

Eucalyptus Tea: Steep dried eucalyptus leaves in hot water to make a soothing herbal tea that can be enjoyed for respiratory support and immune boosting. Eucalyptus tea has a refreshing flavor and can be sweetened with honey for added benefits.

Safety Considerations

While eucalyptus is generally considered safe when used appropriately, it is essential to dilute eucalyptus essential oil properly before applying it to the skin, as it can cause irritation in some individuals. Pregnant or breastfeeding women and young children should consult with a healthcare professional before using eucalyptus oil. Additionally, eucalyptus oil should not be ingested, as it can be toxic in large doses.

Eucalyptus, with its invigorating aroma and potent medicinal properties, offers a natural solution for respiratory congestion, coughs, and colds. Whether inhaled as steam, applied topically as a chest rub, or enjoyed as a soothing tea, eucalyptus provides comfort and relief to those seeking respiratory support. By harnessing the power of eucalyptus, we can breathe easier, stay healthy, and embrace the vitality of nature's pharmacy.

Herbal Remedies for Digestive Health

Introduction

Digestive health plays a crucial role in overall well-being, influencing everything from nutrient absorption to immune function. When the digestive system is out of balance, it can lead to discomfort, bloating, and other digestive issues that impact quality of life. While lifestyle factors such as diet and stress management are essential for maintaining digestive health, herbal remedies offer natural support for promoting optimal digestion and relieving gastrointestinal discomfort. In this chapter, we explore a variety of herbs and herbal preparations that can soothe the digestive system, support gut health, and promote overall digestive wellness.

Understanding Digestive Health

The Importance of Digestive Health: The digestive system is responsible for breaking down food into nutrients, absorbing essential vitamins and minerals, and eliminating waste products from the body. A healthy digestive system is essential for proper nutrient absorption, immune function, and overall vitality.

Common Digestive Issues: Digestive issues can manifest in various forms, including indigestion, bloating, gas, constipation, diarrhea, and acid reflux. These symptoms may be caused by factors such as poor diet, stress, food sensitivities, or imbalances in gut bacteria.

Herbal Remedies for Digestive Health

Peppermint (Mentha piperita):

- Properties: Peppermint has carminative and antispasmodic properties, making it effective for relieving gas, bloating, and stomach cramps.
- Preparation: Drink peppermint tea or chew on fresh peppermint leaves after meals to promote digestion and soothe gastrointestinal discomfort.

Ginger (Zingiber officinale):

- Properties: Ginger is a natural digestive aid, stimulating the production of digestive enzymes and promoting gastric motility.
- Preparation: Drink ginger tea, chew on a piece of fresh ginger, or take ginger supplements to relieve nausea, indigestion, and motion sickness.

Chamomile (Matricaria chamomilla):

- Properties: Chamomile has anti-inflammatory and antispasmodic properties, making it useful for soothing digestive issues such as indigestion, bloating, and abdominal cramps.
- Preparation: Drink chamomile tea before or after meals to promote relaxation, reduce inflammation, and support healthy digestion.

Fennel (Foeniculum vulgare):

- Properties: Fennel seeds contain volatile oils that have carminative and antispasmodic effects, helping to relieve gas, bloating, and stomach cramps.
- Preparation: Chew on fennel seeds after meals or drink fennel tea to aid digestion and alleviate gastrointestinal discomfort.

Dandelion (Taraxacum officinale):

- Properties: Dandelion root is a bitter herb that stimulates bile production and promotes liver and gallbladder health, aiding in digestion and detoxification.
- Preparation: Drink dandelion root tea or take dandelion root supplements to support liver function and improve digestion.

How to Use Herbal Remedies

Herbal Teas: Steep dried herbs in hot water to make soothing herbal teas that can be enjoyed throughout the day to support digestion and relieve gastrointestinal discomfort.

Herbal Tinctures: Take herbal tinctures diluted in water or juice for a concentrated dose of therapeutic benefits. Follow recommended dosage guidelines for each herb.

Herbal Capsules: Take herbal capsules or tablets containing powdered herbs for convenience and ease of use. Follow recommended dosage instructions provided by the manufacturer.

Safety Considerations

While herbal remedies are generally safe when used appropriately, it is essential to consult with a healthcare professional before using herbs, especially if you are pregnant, breastfeeding, or taking medications. Some herbs may interact with medications or exacerbate certain medical conditions.

Herbal remedies offer natural support for promoting digestive health and relieving gastrointestinal discomfort. By incorporating herbs into your daily routine, you can soothe digestive issues, support gut health, and promote overall well-being. Whether enjoyed as a soothing tea, taken as a tincture, or consumed in capsule form, herbal remedies provide gentle and effective relief for common digestive issues. With knowledge and mindfulness, you can harness the power of herbs to support optimal digestion and thrive in harmony with your body.

Ginger: Nature's Digestive Aid

Introduction

Ginger, with its knobby root and distinctive spicy flavor, is not just a staple in culinary traditions around the world but also a powerhouse of medicinal benefits. This versatile herb, scientifically known as Zingiber officinale, has been revered for centuries for its ability to soothe digestive discomfort, alleviate nausea, and promote overall wellness. In this chapter, we explore the remarkable properties of ginger and its role as a natural digestive aid.

Understanding Ginger

Botanical Background: Ginger is a flowering plant belonging to the Zingiberaceae family, native to Southeast Asia but cultivated in many tropical regions worldwide. It is prized for its rhizome, or underground stem, which is harvested for both culinary and medicinal purposes.

Medicinal Properties: Ginger contains bioactive compounds such as gingerol, shogaol, and zingerone, which contribute to its therapeutic effects. These compounds have anti-inflammatory, antioxidant, and antiemetic properties, making ginger highly effective for relieving digestive issues and nausea.

Harnessing the Power of Ginger

Digestive Support: Ginger is perhaps best known for its ability to support digestive health and alleviate gastrointestinal discomfort. It stimulates the production of digestive enzymes, enhances gastric motility, and helps to relieve symptoms such as bloating, gas, and indigestion.

Nausea Relief: Ginger is a natural remedy for nausea and vomiting, whether caused by motion sickness, morning sickness during pregnancy, or chemotherapy. Its antiemetic properties help to calm the stomach and reduce feelings of nausea, making ginger a gentle and effective remedy for queasiness.

Anti-inflammatory Effects: Chronic inflammation in the digestive tract can lead to conditions such as gastritis, acid reflux, and inflammatory bowel disease. Ginger's potent anti-inflammatory properties help to reduce inflammation in the gastrointestinal tract, soothing irritation and promoting healing.

How to Use Ginger

Ginger Tea: Steep fresh or dried ginger slices in hot water to make a soothing ginger tea. Enjoy ginger tea before or after meals to aid digestion, or sip on it throughout the day to relieve nausea and promote overall wellness.

Ginger Chews: Chew on crystallized ginger or ginger candies to alleviate nausea and settle the stomach. Ginger chews are a convenient and portable option for on-the-go relief from digestive discomfort.

Ginger Supplements: Take ginger supplements in capsule or tablet form for a concentrated dose of ginger's therapeutic benefits. Follow recommended dosage guidelines provided by the manufacturer.

Safety Considerations

Ginger is generally considered safe when consumed in moderate amounts, but individuals with certain medical conditions or those taking medications should consult with a healthcare professional before using ginger supplements. Pregnant or breastfeeding women should also exercise caution and avoid consuming excessive amounts of ginger.

Ginger, with its potent medicinal properties and versatile uses, offers a natural solution for digestive issues, nausea, and overall wellness. Whether enjoyed as a soothing tea, chewed as a ginger candy, or taken as a supplement, ginger provides gentle and effective relief for common digestive discomfort. By harnessing the power of ginger, we can support our digestive health, soothe our stomachs, and embrace the healing gifts of nature.

Peppermint: Nature's Digestive Soother

Introduction

Peppermint, with its refreshing scent and cooling taste, holds a special place in both culinary and medicinal traditions. This aromatic herb, scientifically known as Mentha piperita, has been cherished for centuries for its ability to soothe digestive discomfort, alleviate nausea, and promote overall well-being. In this chapter, we explore the remarkable properties of peppermint and its role as a natural digestive aid.

Understanding Peppermint

Botanical Background: Peppermint is a hybrid plant that is a cross between watermint (Mentha aquatica) and spearmint (Mentha spicata). It belongs to the Lamiaceae family and is native to Europe and the Middle East but is now cultivated worldwide for its culinary and medicinal uses.

Medicinal Properties: Peppermint contains several bioactive compounds, including menthol, menthone, and rosmarinic acid, which contribute to its therapeutic effects. These compounds have antispasmodic, carminative, and analgesic properties, making peppermint highly effective for relieving digestive issues and nausea.

Harnessing the Power of Peppermint

Digestive Support: Peppermint is renowned for its ability to support digestive health and alleviate gastrointestinal discomfort. It relaxes the muscles of the digestive tract, reducing spasms and cramping, and helps to relieve symptoms such as bloating, gas, and indigestion.

Nausea Relief: Peppermint is a natural remedy for nausea and vomiting, whether caused by motion sickness, morning sickness during pregnancy, or chemotherapy. Its soothing properties help to calm the stomach and reduce feelings of queasiness, making peppermint a gentle and effective remedy for nausea.

Pain Relief: Peppermint has mild analgesic properties that can help to alleviate digestive pain and discomfort. It acts as a natural pain reliever, reducing inflammation and soothing irritation in the gastrointestinal tract.

How to Use Peppermint

Peppermint Tea: Steep fresh or dried peppermint leaves in hot water to make a soothing peppermint tea. Enjoy peppermint tea before or after meals to aid digestion, or sip on it throughout the day to relieve nausea and promote overall wellness.

Peppermint Oil: Dilute peppermint essential oil in a carrier oil such as coconut or almond oil and apply it topically to the abdomen to relieve digestive discomfort. Peppermint oil can also be added to a warm bath or used in aromatherapy to promote relaxation and soothe the stomach.

Peppermint Supplements: Take peppermint supplements in capsule or tablet form for a concentrated dose of peppermint's therapeutic benefits. Follow recommended dosage guidelines provided by the manufacturer.

Safety Considerations

Peppermint is generally considered safe when consumed in moderate amounts, but individuals with certain medical conditions or those taking medications should consult with a healthcare professional before using peppermint supplements. Pregnant or breastfeeding women should also exercise caution and avoid consuming excessive amounts of peppermint.

Peppermint, with its invigorating aroma and soothing properties, offers a natural solution for digestive issues, nausea, and overall wellness. Whether enjoyed as a soothing tea, applied topically as an oil, or taken as a supplement, peppermint provides gentle and effective relief for common digestive discomfort. By harnessing the power of peppermint, we can support our digestive health, soothe our stomachs, and embrace the healing gifts of nature.

Fennel: Nature's Digestive Comfort

Introduction

Fennel, with its feathery fronds and aromatic seeds, is a culinary and medicinal treasure that has been celebrated for its digestive benefits for centuries. This versatile herb, scientifically known as Foeniculum vulgare, offers a natural solution for digestive discomfort, bloating, and gas. In this chapter, we explore the remarkable properties of fennel and its role as a digestive aid.

Understanding Fennel

Botanical Background: Fennel is a flowering plant belonging to the carrot family, Apiaceae. It is native to the Mediterranean region but is now cultivated in many parts of the world for its culinary and medicinal uses. Fennel is prized for its flavorful seeds, crunchy bulb, and aromatic foliage.

Medicinal Properties: Fennel contains several bioactive compounds, including anethole, fenchone, and estragole, which contribute to its therapeutic effects. These compounds have carminative, antispasmodic, and anti-inflammatory properties, making fennel highly effective for relieving digestive issues and promoting gastrointestinal health.

Harnessing the Power of Fennel

Digestive Support: Fennel is renowned for its ability to support digestive health and alleviate gastrointestinal discomfort. It relaxes the muscles of the digestive tract, reducing spasms and cramping, and helps to relieve symptoms such as bloating, gas, and indigestion.

Gas Relief: Fennel seeds are particularly effective for relieving gas and bloating. Chewing on fennel seeds after meals or drinking fennel tea can help to ease digestive discomfort and reduce flatulence.

Appetite Regulation: Fennel has appetite-suppressing properties and may help to regulate appetite and promote weight loss. Drinking fennel tea between meals can help to curb cravings and support healthy eating habits.

How to Use Fennel

Fennel Tea: Steep crushed fennel seeds in hot water to make a soothing fennel tea. Enjoy fennel tea before or after meals to aid digestion, or sip on it throughout the day to relieve gas and bloating.

Fennel Seeds: Chew on a small handful of fennel seeds after meals to promote digestion and freshen breath. Fennel seeds can also be added to culinary dishes such as soups, stews, and salads for flavor and digestive support.

Fennel Oil: Dilute fennel essential oil in a carrier oil such as coconut or olive oil and massage it onto the abdomen to relieve digestive discomfort. Fennel oil can also be diffused aromatically to promote relaxation and soothe the stomach.

Safety Considerations

Fennel is generally considered safe when consumed in moderate amounts, but individuals with certain medical conditions or those taking medications should consult with a healthcare professional before using fennel supplements. Pregnant or breastfeeding women should also exercise caution and avoid consuming excessive amounts of fennel.

Fennel, with its aromatic seeds and digestive benefits, offers a natural solution for gastrointestinal discomfort and bloating. Whether enjoyed as a soothing tea, chewed as seeds, or applied topically as an oil, fennel provides gentle and effective relief for common digestive issues. By incorporating the power of fennel into our daily lives, we can support digestive health, soothe discomfort, and embrace the healing gifts of nature.

Chamomile: Nature's Digestive Comforter

Introduction

Chamomile, with its delicate flowers and soothing aroma, has long been cherished for its calming properties and its ability to promote digestive health. This gentle herb, scientifically known as Matricaria chamomilla or Chamaemelum nobile, offers a natural solution for soothing digestive discomfort, relieving indigestion, and promoting overall well-being. In this chapter, we explore the remarkable properties of chamomile and its role as a digestive aid.

Understanding Chamomile

Botanical Background: Chamomile is a flowering plant belonging to the Asteraceae family. There are two primary species of chamomile used for medicinal purposes: German chamomile (Matricaria chamomilla) and Roman or English chamomile (Chamaemelum nobile). Both varieties have similar medicinal properties and are valued for their calming effects.

Medicinal Properties: Chamomile contains several bioactive compounds, including chamazulene, apigenin, and bisabolol, which contribute to its therapeutic effects. These compounds have anti-inflammatory, antispasmodic, and carminative properties, making chamomile highly effective for relieving digestive issues and promoting gastrointestinal health.

Harnessing the Power of Chamomile

Digestive Support: Chamomile is renowned for its ability to support digestive health and alleviate gastrointestinal discomfort. It relaxes the muscles of the digestive tract, reducing spasms and cramping, and helps to relieve symptoms such as bloating, gas, and indigestion.

Indigestion Relief: Chamomile tea is particularly effective for relieving indigestion and heartburn. Drinking chamomile tea before or after meals can help to soothe the stomach, reduce acidity, and promote digestion.

Stress Reduction: Chamomile has natural calming properties that help to reduce stress and anxiety, which can contribute to digestive issues. Drinking chamomile tea regularly can help to promote relaxation, improve mood, and support overall well-being.

How to Use Chamomile

Chamomile Tea: Steep dried chamomile flowers in hot water to make a soothing chamomile tea. Enjoy chamomile tea before or after meals to aid digestion, or sip on it throughout the day to promote relaxation and reduce stress.

Chamomile Supplements: Take chamomile supplements in capsule or tablet form for a concentrated dose of chamomile's therapeutic benefits. Follow recommended dosage guidelines provided by the manufacturer.

Chamomile Essential Oil: Dilute chamomile essential oil in a carrier oil such as coconut or almond oil and massage it onto the abdomen to relieve digestive discomfort. Chamomile oil can also be diffused aromatically to promote relaxation and soothe the stomach.

Safety Considerations

Chamomile is generally considered safe when consumed in moderate amounts, but individuals with certain medical conditions or those taking medications should consult with a healthcare professional before using chamomile supplements. Pregnant or breastfeeding women should also exercise caution and avoid consuming excessive amounts of chamomile.

Chamomile, with its gentle nature and calming effects, offers a natural solution for digestive discomfort and stress. Whether enjoyed as a soothing tea, taken as a supplement, or applied topically as an oil, chamomile provides gentle and effective relief for common digestive issues. By incorporating the power of chamomile into our daily lives, we can support digestive health, reduce stress, and embrace the healing gifts of nature.

Immune System Support: Harnessing Nature's Defense

Introduction

The immune system serves as the body's primary defense against pathogens, helping to ward off infections and maintain overall health. While a balanced diet, regular exercise, and adequate sleep are key pillars of immune health, certain herbs and natural remedies can provide additional support. In this chapter, we explore a variety of herbs and botanicals renowned for their immune-boosting properties, helping to fortify the body's natural defenses and promote resilience against illness.

Understanding Immune System Support

The Importance of Immune Health: The immune system plays a vital role in protecting the body against harmful invaders, including bacteria, viruses, and other pathogens. A robust immune system is essential for maintaining overall health, preventing infections, and supporting timely recovery.

Common Immune Challenges: Factors such as stress, poor nutrition, lack of sleep, and environmental toxins can compromise immune function, making individuals more susceptible to infections and illnesses. Supporting immune health through lifestyle choices and natural remedies can help to bolster the body's defenses and enhance resilience.

Herbs for Immune Support

Echinacea (Echinacea purpurea):

- Properties: Echinacea is renowned for its immune-boosting properties, stimulating the production of white blood cells and enhancing the body's natural defense mechanisms.
- Preparation: Take echinacea supplements or drink echinacea tea at the onset of illness to support immune function and promote faster recovery.

Elderberry (Sambucus nigra):

- Properties: Elderberry is rich in antioxidants and vitamins that help to strengthen the immune system and protect against respiratory infections.
- Preparation: Take elderberry syrup or elderberry supplements daily during cold and flu season to support immune health and reduce the severity of symptoms.

Astragalus (Astragalus membranaceus):

- Properties: Astragalus is an adaptogenic herb that supports immune function by modulating the body's response to stress and enhancing immune cell activity.
- Preparation: Take astragalus supplements or drink astragalus tea regularly to support immune health and promote overall well-being.

Garlic (Allium sativum):

- Properties: Garlic contains compounds such as allicin, which have antimicrobial and immune-boosting properties, helping to ward off infections and support immune function.
- Preparation: Incorporate fresh garlic into culinary dishes or take garlic supplements to support immune health and promote cardiovascular health.

Ginger (Zingiber officinale):

- Properties: Ginger has anti-inflammatory and antioxidant properties that help to support immune function and reduce inflammation in the body.
- Preparation: Drink ginger tea or use fresh ginger in culinary dishes to promote immune health and alleviate symptoms of illness.

How to Use Immune-Boosting Herbs

Herbal Teas: Steep dried herbs in hot water to make immune-boosting herbal teas that can be enjoyed throughout the day to support immune function and promote overall well-being.

Herbal Supplements: Take herbal supplements in capsule or tablet form for a concentrated dose of immune-boosting herbs. Follow recommended dosage guidelines provided by the manufacturer.

Herbal Tinctures: Take herbal tinctures diluted in water or juice for a convenient and effective way to support immune health. Follow recommended dosage instructions provided by the manufacturer.

Safety Considerations

While herbs are generally safe when used appropriately, it is essential to consult with a healthcare professional before using herbal supplements, especially if you are pregnant, breastfeeding, or taking medications. Some herbs may interact with medications or exacerbate certain medical conditions.

Immune system support is essential for maintaining overall health and resilience against illness. By incorporating immune-boosting herbs into your daily routine, you can strengthen your body's natural defenses, reduce the risk of infections, and promote overall well-being. With knowledge and mindfulness, you can harness the power of nature to support immune health and thrive in harmony with your body.

Echinacea: Nature's Immune Booster

Introduction

Echinacea, with its vibrant petals and robust roots, has earned a well-deserved reputation as a potent immune-boosting herb. Scientifically known as Echinacea purpurea or Echinacea angustifolia, this remarkable plant has been used for centuries by indigenous cultures for its ability to support immune health and promote overall well-being. In this chapter, we delve into the rich history and powerful properties of echinacea as a natural ally in fortifying the body's defenses against illness.

Understanding Echinacea

Botanical Background: Echinacea is a genus of flowering plants in the daisy family, Asteraceae, native to North America. It is characterized by its striking purple, pink, or white petals and prominent cone-shaped seed head. Echinacea species, including Echinacea purpurea and Echinacea angustifolia, have long been valued for their medicinal properties.

Medicinal Properties: Echinacea contains a variety of bioactive compounds, including alkamides, polysaccharides, and flavonoids, which contribute to its immune-boosting effects. These compounds help to stimulate the production and activity of white blood cells, enhancing the body's ability to fight off infections and pathogens.

Harnessing the Power of Echinacea

Immune Support: Echinacea is renowned for its ability to support immune function and promote resilience against illness. It stimulates the production of white blood cells, including T-cells and macrophages, which play a crucial role in the body's defense against infections.

Cold and Flu Relief: Echinacea is often used to reduce the severity and duration of colds, flu, and other respiratory infections. Taking echinacea supplements or drinking echinacea tea at the onset of illness can help to boost the immune response and promote faster recovery.

Wound Healing: Echinacea has antiseptic and anti-inflammatory properties that make it beneficial for promoting wound healing and reducing the risk of infection. Applying echinacea tincture or ointment topically to cuts, scrapes, and minor wounds can help to accelerate the healing process.

How to Use Echinacea

Echinacea Tea: Steep dried echinacea roots, leaves, or flowers in hot water to make a soothing echinacea tea. Enjoy echinacea tea regularly during cold and flu season to support immune health and reduce the risk of infections.

Echinacea Supplements: Take echinacea supplements in capsule, tablet, or tincture form for a concentrated dose of immune-boosting benefits. Follow recommended dosage guidelines provided by the manufacturer.

Echinacea Tincture: Take echinacea tincture diluted in water or juice for a convenient and effective way to support immune health. Follow recommended dosage instructions provided by the manufacturer.

Safety Considerations

Echinacea is generally safe for most people when used appropriately, but individuals with certain medical conditions or those taking immunosuppressant medications should consult with a healthcare professional before using echinacea supplements. Pregnant or breastfeeding women should also exercise caution and avoid consuming excessive amounts of echinacea.

Echinacea, with its immune-boosting properties and long history of use in traditional medicine, offers a natural solution for promoting immune health and resilience against illness. Whether enjoyed as a soothing tea, taken as a supplement, or applied topically as a tincture, echinacea provides gentle and effective support for the body's defenses. By harnessing the power of echinacea, we can strengthen our immune system, reduce the risk of infections, and embrace the healing gifts of nature.

Astragalus: Nature's Immune Modulator

Introduction

Astragalus, with its resilient roots and delicate flowers, has long been revered in traditional Chinese medicine for its powerful immune-modulating properties. Scientifically known as Astragalus membranaceus, this remarkable herb offers a natural solution for strengthening the immune system, enhancing vitality, and promoting overall well-being. In this chapter, we delve into the fascinating properties of astragalus and its role as a potent immune supporter.

Understanding Astragalus

Botanical Background: Astragalus is a perennial herbaceous plant belonging to the Fabaceae family, native to the temperate regions of Asia. It is characterized by its hairy stems, pinnate leaves, and clusters of small yellow flowers. Astragalus root, known as Huang Qi in traditional Chinese medicine, has been used for thousands of years for its medicinal properties.

Medicinal Properties: Astragalus root contains a variety of bioactive compounds, including polysaccharides, saponins, and flavonoids, which contribute to its immune-boosting effects. These compounds help to modulate the immune system, enhancing the body's ability to fight off infections and maintain optimal health.

Harnessing the Power of Astragalus

Immune Support: Astragalus is renowned for its ability to support immune function and promote resilience against infections. It stimulates the production of white blood cells, including T-cells and macrophages, which play a crucial role in the body's defense against pathogens.

Adaptogenic Properties: Astragalus is an adaptogenic herb, meaning it helps the body adapt to stress and maintain balance. By modulating the body's stress response, astragalus supports immune health and promotes overall well-being.

Anti-inflammatory Effects: Astragalus has anti-inflammatory properties that help to reduce inflammation in the body and support immune function. It helps to calm inflammation in the respiratory tract, soothe coughs, and promote faster recovery from respiratory illnesses.

How to Use Astragalus

Astragalus Supplements: Take astragalus supplements in capsule or tablet form for a concentrated dose of immune-boosting benefits. Follow recommended dosage guidelines provided by the manufacturer.

Astragalus Tea: Steep dried astragalus root slices in hot water to make a soothing astragalus tea. Enjoy astragalus tea regularly as a warm and comforting beverage that supports immune health and promotes overall wellness.

Astragalus Tincture: Take astragalus tincture diluted in water or juice for a convenient and effective way to support immune health. Follow recommended dosage instructions provided by the manufacturer.

Safety Considerations

Astragalus is generally safe for most people when used appropriately, but individuals with certain medical conditions or those taking immunosuppressant medications should consult with a healthcare professional before using astragalus supplements. Pregnant or breastfeeding women should also exercise caution and avoid consuming excessive amounts of astragalus.

Astragalus, with its immune-modulating properties and long history of use in traditional medicine, offers a natural solution for promoting immune health and resilience against infections. Whether enjoyed as a supplement, brewed into a soothing tea, or taken as a tincture, astragalus provides gentle and effective support for the body's defenses. By harnessing the power of astragalus, we can strengthen our immune system, reduce the risk of infections, and embrace the healing gifts of nature.

Garlic: Nature's Potent Immune Booster

Introduction

Garlic, with its pungent aroma and robust flavor, has been cherished for centuries not only as a culinary staple but also as a powerful medicinal herb. Scientifically known as Allium sativum, garlic offers a wealth of health benefits, particularly in bolstering the immune system and promoting overall well-being. In this chapter, we explore the remarkable properties of garlic and its role as a natural immune booster.

Understanding Garlic

Botanical Background: Garlic is a member of the Allium genus, which also includes onions, leeks, and shallots. It is characterized by its distinctive bulb composed of multiple cloves encased in a papery skin. Garlic has been cultivated for thousands of years and is widely used in cuisines around the world.

Medicinal Properties: Garlic contains several bioactive compounds, including allicin, diallyl sulfide, and saponins, which contribute to its medicinal properties. These compounds have antimicrobial, antioxidant, and immune-boosting effects, making garlic a potent ally in promoting health and wellness.

Harnessing the Power of Garlic

Immune Support: Garlic is renowned for its ability to support immune function and enhance the body's natural defenses against infections. It stimulates the production of white blood cells, including T-cells and macrophages, which play a crucial role in the immune response.

Antimicrobial Activity: Garlic has potent antimicrobial properties that help to fight off bacteria, viruses, fungi, and parasites. It can help to prevent and alleviate various infections, including colds, flu, and respiratory illnesses.

Anti-inflammatory Effects: Garlic has anti-inflammatory properties that help to reduce inflammation in the body and support immune function. It can help to alleviate symptoms of inflammatory conditions and promote overall well-being.

How to Use Garlic

Raw Garlic: Consuming raw garlic is one of the most potent ways to harness its immune-boosting benefits. Crush or mince garlic cloves and let them sit for a few minutes to activate the beneficial compounds, then add them to salads, dressings, or other culinary dishes.

Garlic Supplements: Take garlic supplements in capsule or tablet form for a concentrated dose of immune-boosting benefits. Follow recommended dosage guidelines provided by the manufacturer.

Garlic Oil: Use garlic oil topically to promote wound healing and prevent infections. Dilute garlic oil in a carrier oil such as olive or coconut oil and apply it to cuts, scrapes, or other skin irritations.

Safety Considerations

Garlic is generally safe for most people when consumed in moderate amounts as a food ingredient. However, individuals with certain medical conditions, such as bleeding disorders or gastrointestinal issues, should exercise caution when consuming garlic supplements. Pregnant or breastfeeding women should also consult with a healthcare professional before using garlic supplements.

Garlic, with its potent immune-boosting and antimicrobial properties, offers a natural solution for promoting immune health and warding off infections. Whether enjoyed raw in culinary dishes or taken as a supplement, garlic provides gentle and effective support for the body's defenses. By incorporating garlic into our daily lives, we can strengthen our immune system, reduce the risk of infections, and embrace the healing gifts of nature.

Understanding Skin Conditions: A Holistic Approach to Dermatological Health

Introduction

Skin, the largest organ of the human body, serves as a protective barrier against external threats while also reflecting internal health. Dermatological conditions, ranging from minor irritations to chronic disorders, can significantly impact quality of life. In this chapter, we explore the multifaceted nature of skin health, discussing common conditions, underlying causes, and holistic approaches to support dermatological well-being.

Exploring Skin Conditions

Common Dermatological Conditions: Skin conditions encompass a broad spectrum, including acne, eczema, psoriasis, rosacea, dermatitis, and fungal infections. These conditions vary in severity, symptoms, and triggers, but all can affect physical comfort, self-esteem, and overall health.

Underlying Factors: Dermatological conditions often arise from a combination of genetic predisposition, environmental factors, lifestyle choices, and immune system dysregulation. Triggers such as stress, hormonal fluctuations, dietary factors, allergens, pollutants, and microbial imbalances can exacerbate symptoms.

Holistic Approaches to Skin Health

Nutritional Support: A balanced diet rich in vitamins, minerals, antioxidants, and essential fatty acids supports skin health from within. Incorporating foods such as fruits, vegetables, whole grains, lean proteins, and healthy fats nourishes the skin and promotes optimal function.

Stress Management: Chronic stress can exacerbate skin conditions by triggering inflammation, hormonal imbalances, and immune system dysfunction. Practices such as mindfulness, meditation, yoga, deep breathing exercises, and adequate sleep promote relaxation and support skin health.

Topical Treatments: Natural remedies such as aloe vera, coconut oil, tea tree oil, calendula, chamomile, and oatmeal can soothe irritated skin, reduce inflammation, and support healing. Choosing gentle, non-toxic skincare products free of harsh chemicals and irritants is essential for maintaining skin health.

Hydration: Adequate hydration is vital for skin health, as it helps to maintain moisture balance, support elasticity, and facilitate detoxification. Drinking plenty of water and using hydrating skincare products help to keep the skin supple, smooth, and resilient.

Sun Protection: Protecting the skin from harmful UV radiation is crucial for preventing premature aging, sunburn, and skin cancer. Using broad-spectrum sunscreen, wearing protective clothing, seeking shade, and avoiding excessive sun exposure help to safeguard skin health.

Collaborative Care

Consultation with Healthcare Professionals: Seeking guidance from dermatologists, naturopathic doctors, or other healthcare providers specializing in skin health is essential for accurate diagnosis and personalized treatment plans. Integrating conventional and complementary approaches ensures comprehensive care and optimal outcomes.

Self-Care and Empowerment: Empowering individuals to take an active role in their skin health through education, self-care practices, and lifestyle modifications fosters a sense of control and resilience. Mindful skincare routines, stress management techniques, and dietary modifications support long-term dermatological well-being.

Skin conditions, while diverse and complex, can be effectively managed and supported through holistic approaches that address underlying factors and promote overall health and well-being. By adopting a multidimensional perspective that considers nutritional support, stress management, topical treatments, hydration, sun protection, and collaborative care, individuals can nurture healthy, radiant skin and embrace the beauty of holistic dermatological health.

Aloe Vera: Nature's Soothing Skin Healer

Introduction

Aloe vera, with its succulent leaves and cooling gel, has been treasured for centuries for its remarkable healing properties. Scientifically known as Aloe barbadensis miller, this versatile plant offers a natural solution for a wide range of skin conditions, from minor irritations to more serious concerns. In this chapter, we explore the extraordinary benefits of aloe vera and its role as a soothing skin healer.

Understanding Aloe Vera

Botanical Background: Aloe vera is a perennial succulent plant that belongs to the Asphodelaceae family. Native to the Arabian Peninsula, aloe vera is now cultivated worldwide for its medicinal and cosmetic uses. It is characterized by its fleshy, spear-shaped leaves that contain a gel-like substance.

Medicinal Properties: Aloe vera gel contains a complex mixture of bioactive compounds, including polysaccharides, vitamins, minerals, amino acids, and antioxidants. These compounds have anti-inflammatory, antimicrobial, and wound-healing properties, making aloe vera an effective remedy for various skin conditions.

Harnessing the Power of Aloe Vera

Skin Healing: Aloe vera gel is renowned for its ability to promote wound healing and tissue regeneration. It accelerates the healing process by reducing inflammation, stimulating cell proliferation, and enhancing collagen production, resulting in faster recovery from cuts, burns, and abrasions.

Soothing Irritations: Aloe vera gel has a cooling and hydrating effect on the skin, making it ideal for soothing irritations such as sunburn, rashes, insect bites, and allergic reactions. It helps to alleviate pain, reduce redness, and restore moisture balance to the skin.

Moisturizing: Aloe vera gel acts as a natural moisturizer, penetrating deep into the skin to hydrate and nourish from within. It softens the skin, improves elasticity, and promotes a healthy, radiant complexion without clogging pores or leaving a greasy residue.

How to Use Aloe Vera

Topical Application: Apply pure aloe vera gel directly to the affected area of the skin, gently massaging it in until absorbed. Repeat as needed to soothe irritation, promote healing, and maintain skin health.

DIY Skincare Products: Incorporate aloe vera gel into homemade skincare recipes such as face masks, moisturizers, and serums for a natural boost of hydration and healing properties.

Commercial Products: Choose skincare products containing high-quality aloe vera gel as a key ingredient, such as lotions, creams, gels, and sunscreens, to benefit from its soothing and moisturizing effects.

Safety Considerations

Aloe vera is generally safe for most people when used topically, but individuals with sensitive skin or allergies may experience irritation or allergic reactions. It is advisable to perform a patch test before using aloe vera products extensively, especially if you have known sensitivities. Internal use of aloe vera, such as consuming aloe vera juice, should be done with caution and under the guidance of a healthcare professional, as it may cause gastrointestinal discomfort in some individuals.

Aloe vera, with its soothing gel and healing properties, offers a natural solution for a variety of skin concerns. Whether used to accelerate wound healing, soothe irritations, or moisturize the skin, aloe vera provides gentle and effective care for healthy, radiant skin. By harnessing the power of aloe vera, we can nurture our skin and embrace the healing gifts of nature.

Calendula: Nature's Gentle Skin Healer

Introduction

Calendula, with its vibrant orange or yellow flowers and myriad medicinal properties, has been revered for centuries as a healing herb. Scientifically known as Calendula officinalis, this versatile plant offers a natural solution for a wide range of skin ailments, from minor irritations to more serious conditions. In this chapter, we explore the extraordinary benefits of calendula and its role as a gentle skin healer.

Understanding Calendula

Botanical Background: Calendula is a member of the Asteraceae family, native to the Mediterranean region but now cultivated worldwide for its medicinal and ornamental value. It is characterized by its bright, daisy-like flowers that bloom profusely throughout the growing season.

Medicinal Properties: Calendula flowers contain a rich array of bioactive compounds, including flavonoids, saponins, and triterpenoids, which contribute to its healing properties. These compounds have anti-inflammatory, antimicrobial, and wound-healing effects, making calendula an effective remedy for various skin conditions.

Harnessing the Power of Calendula

Skin Healing: Calendula is renowned for its ability to promote wound healing and tissue regeneration. It accelerates the healing process by reducing inflammation, promoting cell proliferation, and enhancing collagen synthesis, resulting in faster recovery from cuts, burns, and abrasions.

Soothing Irritations: Calendula has a gentle and calming effect on the skin, making it ideal for soothing irritations such as sunburn, rashes, eczema, and dermatitis. It helps to alleviate itching, reduce redness, and restore the skin's natural barrier function.

Anti-inflammatory Action: Calendula possesses potent anti-inflammatory properties that help to calm inflammation and irritation in the skin. It can be used to alleviate symptoms of inflammatory skin conditions such as acne, rosacea, and psoriasis, promoting overall skin health and comfort.

How to Use Calendula

Topical Application: Apply calendula-infused oil, cream, or ointment directly to the affected area of the skin, gently massaging it in until absorbed. Repeat as needed to soothe irritation, promote healing, and maintain skin health.

Calendula Tea: Brew dried calendula flowers into a soothing tea, allowing it to cool before applying it to the skin with a clean cloth or cotton pad. Calendula tea can be used as a gentle toner or compress to soothe inflamed or irritated skin.

Commercial Products: Choose skincare products containing calendula extract or oil as a key ingredient, such as lotions, creams, balms, and salves, to benefit from its healing and soothing properties.

Safety Considerations

Calendula is generally safe for most people when used topically, but individuals with sensitive skin or allergies may experience irritation or allergic reactions. It is advisable to perform a patch test before using calendula products extensively, especially if you have known sensitivities.

Calendula, with its gentle nature and potent healing properties, offers a natural solution for a variety of skin concerns. Whether used to accelerate wound healing, soothe irritations, or calm inflammation, calendula provides gentle and effective care for healthy, radiant skin. By harnessing the power of calendula, we can nurture our skin and embrace the healing gifts of nature.

Tea Tree Oil: Nature's Potent Antimicrobial

Introduction

Tea tree oil, with its fresh, camphoraceous scent and powerful antimicrobial properties, has long been revered as a natural remedy for various skin conditions. Derived from the leaves of the tea tree (Melaleuca alternifolia), this essential oil offers a wide range of therapeutic benefits, making it a staple in aromatherapy and skincare. In this chapter, we explore the remarkable properties of tea tree oil and its role as a potent antimicrobial agent.

Understanding Tea Tree Oil

Botanical Background: Tea tree oil is extracted from the leaves of the tea tree, a small evergreen tree native to Australia. Indigenous Australian communities have used tea tree leaves for centuries to treat wounds, infections, and skin ailments, recognizing their potent healing properties.

Medicinal Properties: Tea tree oil contains a variety of bioactive compounds, including terpinen-4-ol, cineole, and alpha-pinene, which contribute to its antimicrobial, anti-inflammatory, and antiseptic effects. These compounds make tea tree oil highly effective in combating bacteria, fungi, and viruses.

Harnessing the Power of Tea Tree Oil

Antimicrobial Action: Tea tree oil is renowned for its broad-spectrum antimicrobial activity, making it effective against a wide range of pathogens, including bacteria, fungi, and viruses. It inhibits the growth and spread of microorganisms, making it an invaluable tool for treating infections and promoting wound healing.

Acne Treatment: Tea tree oil is a popular natural remedy for acne due to its antimicrobial and anti-inflammatory properties. It helps to kill acne-causing bacteria, reduce inflammation, and unclog pores, resulting in clearer, healthier skin without the side effects associated with conventional acne treatments.

Skin Care: Tea tree oil is widely used in skincare products such as cleansers, toners, and serums for its purifying and clarifying properties. It helps to balance oil production, reduce blemishes, and promote a clearer, more radiant complexion.

How to Use Tea Tree Oil

Topical Application: Dilute tea tree oil with a carrier oil such as coconut oil or jojoba oil before applying it to the skin to avoid irritation. Apply a small amount of diluted tea tree oil to the affected area using a cotton swab or clean fingertips. Repeat as needed to treat infections, acne, or other skin concerns.

Aromatherapy: Add a few drops of tea tree oil to a diffuser or steaming bowl of water to enjoy its purifying and invigorating aroma. Tea tree oil can help to cleanse the air, promote respiratory health, and uplift the mood.

Hair Care: Incorporate tea tree oil into your hair care routine by adding a few drops to your shampoo or conditioner. Tea tree oil helps to control dandruff, soothe scalp irritation, and promote healthy hair growth.

Safety Considerations

Tea tree oil is generally safe for most people when used topically in diluted form. However, undiluted tea tree oil may cause skin irritation or allergic reactions in some individuals, especially those with sensitive skin. It is essential to perform a patch test before using tea tree oil extensively and to dilute it properly with a carrier oil. Internal use of tea tree oil is not recommended, as it can be toxic if ingested.

Tea tree oil, with its potent antimicrobial properties and versatile applications, offers a natural solution for a variety of skin and hair concerns. Whether used to treat infections, combat acne, or promote overall skin health, tea tree oil provides gentle and effective care rooted in nature. By harnessing the power of tea tree oil, we can support our skin and hair health while embracing the healing gifts of the natural world.

Lavender: Nature's Calming Elixir

Introduction

Lavender, with its delicate purple blossoms and sweet floral aroma, has been cherished for centuries for its calming and healing properties. Scientifically known as Lavandula angustifolia, this versatile herb offers a wide range of therapeutic benefits, making it a staple in aromatherapy, skincare, and holistic medicine. In this chapter, we explore the extraordinary properties of lavender and its role as a natural remedy for relaxation and well-being.

Understanding Lavender

Botanical Background: Lavender is a member of the Lamiaceae family, native to the Mediterranean region but now cultivated worldwide for its fragrant flowers and aromatic leaves. Lavender has a long history of use in traditional medicine, culinary arts, and perfumery, dating back thousands of years.

Medicinal Properties: Lavender contains a complex mixture of bioactive compounds, including linalool, linalyl acetate, and camphor, which contribute to its calming, anti-inflammatory, and antiseptic effects. These compounds make lavender oil highly versatile and effective in promoting relaxation, soothing skin irritations, and supporting overall well-being.

Harnessing the Power of Lavender

Relaxation and Stress Relief: Lavender is renowned for its ability to promote relaxation and reduce stress. Its soothing aroma helps to calm the mind, alleviate anxiety, and improve sleep quality, making it an invaluable tool for relaxation and self-care.

Skin Care: Lavender oil is widely used in skincare products such as lotions, creams, and balms for its soothing and healing properties. It helps to moisturize the skin, reduce inflammation, and promote wound healing, making it suitable for various skin concerns, including burns, cuts, insect bites, and acne.

Aromatherapy: Lavender oil is a popular choice for aromatherapy due to its calming and uplifting fragrance. It can be diffused in the air, added to bathwater, or applied topically to pulse points for relaxation, stress relief, and mood enhancement.

How to Use Lavender

Aromatherapy: Add a few drops of lavender oil to a diffuser or steaming bowl of water to enjoy its calming aroma. Lavender oil can help to create a peaceful and tranquil atmosphere, promote relaxation, and improve sleep quality.

Topical Application: Dilute lavender oil with a carrier oil such as coconut oil or almond oil before applying it to the skin. Lavender oil can be applied directly to the skin to soothe minor irritations, relieve muscle tension, or promote relaxation.

Bath: Add a few drops of lavender oil to a warm bath for a relaxing and rejuvenating experience. Lavender-scented baths help to soothe sore muscles, reduce stress, and promote a sense of well-being.

Safety Considerations

Lavender oil is generally safe for most people when used topically or aromatically, but individuals with sensitive skin may experience irritation or allergic reactions. It is essential to perform a patch test before using lavender oil extensively and to dilute it properly with a carrier oil. Internal use of lavender oil is not recommended, as it can be toxic if ingested.

Lavender, with its calming aroma and healing properties, offers a natural solution for relaxation, stress relief, and overall well-being. Whether enjoyed through aromatherapy, applied topically to the skin, or added to bathwater, lavender provides gentle and effective care rooted in nature. By harnessing the power of lavender, we can create moments of tranquility, promote relaxation, and embrace the healing gifts of the natural world.

Introduction: Herbal Solutions for Chronic Conditions

In the realm of healthcare, the pursuit of remedies for chronic conditions often leads us to explore the vast landscape of herbal medicine. Across cultures and throughout history, herbal remedies have been valued for their efficacy, accessibility, and holistic approach to healing. In this exploration, we embark on a journey to uncover the profound potential of herbs in addressing chronic conditions.

Chronic conditions, ranging from autoimmune disorders to cardiovascular diseases, present complex challenges that conventional medicine often struggles to fully alleviate. Yet, within the rich tapestry of nature, there exists a treasure trove of botanical allies offering relief, restoration, and renewal. Herbal solutions, rooted in centuries of traditional wisdom and supported by modern scientific research, hold promise in complementing conventional treatments and enhancing overall well-being.

In this chapter, we delve into the fascinating world of herbal medicine, exploring the mechanisms of action, evidence-based research, and practical applications of herbs in managing chronic conditions. From adaptogenic herbs that support resilience to anti-inflammatory botanicals that soothe discomfort, each herb offers a unique profile of bioactive compounds and therapeutic benefits.

As we navigate through the pages ahead, we invite you to embark on a journey of discovery, empowerment, and healing. Together, let us explore the intricate synergy between humans and herbs, unlocking the potential for profound transformation in the management of chronic conditions. Through knowledge, compassion, and the wisdom of nature, we pave the way towards a future where herbal solutions play a vital role in promoting health, vitality, and resilience for all.

Herbal Relief for Arthritis and Joint Pain

Arthritis and joint pain, pervasive and often debilitating, stand as formidable adversaries in the quest for mobility and comfort. From osteoarthritis, the wear and tear of aging, to rheumatoid arthritis, an autoimmune assault on the joints, these conditions impose significant challenges on those affected. While conventional treatments offer relief for some, others seek alternative approaches rooted in nature's pharmacopeia. In this chapter, we explore herbal remedies for arthritis and joint pain, offering solace and support through botanical allies.

Understanding Arthritis and Joint Pain

Arthritis, a term encompassing a spectrum of inflammatory joint disorders, manifests in various forms, each presenting its unique set of challenges. Osteoarthritis, characterized by the breakdown of cartilage and bone, results in pain, stiffness, and reduced mobility. Rheumatoid arthritis, an autoimmune condition, triggers inflammation, swelling, and joint damage, leading to chronic pain and disability.

Herbal Solutions

Turmeric: Renowned for its potent anti-inflammatory properties, turmeric, with its active compound curcumin, offers relief from arthritis pain and inflammation. Studies suggest that turmeric may inhibit inflammatory pathways, reduce joint swelling, and improve overall joint function.

Ginger: A versatile herb with analgesic and anti-inflammatory effects, ginger provides relief from arthritis pain and stiffness. Its bioactive compounds, including gingerol and shogaol, help to reduce inflammation, alleviate discomfort, and improve joint mobility.

Boswellia: Also known as Indian frankincense, boswellia resin contains boswellic acids, which possess anti-inflammatory and analgesic properties. Boswellia extract has been shown to reduce inflammation in the joints, improve mobility, and alleviate arthritis symptoms.

Devil's Claw: Traditionally used to treat arthritis and other inflammatory conditions, devil's claw contains iridoid glycosides, which exhibit anti-inflammatory and analgesic effects. Devil's claw may help to reduce pain, inflammation, and stiffness associated with arthritis.

Application and Considerations

Herbal remedies for arthritis and joint pain can be consumed as supplements, brewed into teas, or applied topically as ointments or poultices. It is essential to consult with a healthcare professional before incorporating herbal treatments into your arthritis management plan, especially if you are taking medications or have underlying health conditions.

Arthritis and joint pain need not be insurmountable obstacles on the journey to wellness. Through the gentle yet potent interventions of herbal medicine, relief and restoration are within reach. By harnessing the power of nature's botanical allies, we can ease discomfort, promote mobility, and reclaim the joy of movement in our lives.

Turmeric: Nature's Golden Remedy

Introduction

Turmeric, with its vibrant golden hue and centuries-old legacy, stands as a beacon of healing in the realm of herbal medicine. Revered for its potent anti-inflammatory and antioxidant properties, this ancient spice has transcended culinary borders to become a cornerstone of natural health and wellness. In this chapter, we explore the extraordinary benefits of turmeric and its role as a powerhouse remedy for a myriad of health concerns.

Understanding Turmeric

Botanical Background: Turmeric, scientifically known as Curcuma longa, is a perennial herbaceous plant belonging to the ginger family, native to South Asia. It is cultivated for its rhizomes, which are dried and ground into the golden powder we know as turmeric.

Medicinal Properties: Turmeric owes its healing prowess to its primary bioactive compound, curcumin. Curcumin is a potent antioxidant and anti-inflammatory agent, offering a wide range of therapeutic benefits for various health conditions.

Harnessing the Power of Turmeric

Anti-inflammatory Action: Turmeric's most celebrated attribute is its ability to quell inflammation throughout the body. Curcumin inhibits inflammatory pathways, reducing inflammation at the molecular level and providing relief for conditions such as arthritis, inflammatory bowel disease, and chronic pain.

Antioxidant Protection: Turmeric boasts powerful antioxidant properties that help neutralize harmful free radicals and protect cells from oxidative damage. This antioxidant activity supports overall health and may help prevent chronic diseases associated with oxidative stress, such as heart disease, cancer, and neurodegenerative disorders.

Digestive Support: Turmeric aids digestion and promotes gastrointestinal health by stimulating bile production, supporting liver function, and soothing inflammation in the digestive tract. It may help alleviate symptoms of indigestion, bloating, and irritable bowel syndrome (IBS).

How to Use Turmeric

Golden Milk: Prepare a soothing and nutritious golden milk by simmering turmeric powder with milk (or a dairy-free alternative), black pepper, and other warming spices such as cinnamon and ginger. Enjoy this comforting beverage as a bedtime ritual or a midday pick-me-up.

Curcumin Supplements: Take curcumin supplements in capsule or tablet form for a concentrated dose of turmeric's therapeutic benefits. Look for supplements that contain piperine, a compound found in black pepper that enhances curcumin absorption.

Culinary Delight: Incorporate turmeric powder into your culinary creations to add flavor and color while reaping its health benefits. Sprinkle turmeric onto roasted vegetables, soups, stews, curries, and smoothies for a nutritional boost.

Safety Considerations

Turmeric is generally safe for most people when consumed in culinary amounts or taken as a supplement. However, high doses of turmeric may cause gastrointestinal discomfort or interact with certain medications. Consult with a healthcare professional before using turmeric supplements, especially if you are pregnant, breastfeeding, or taking blood-thinning medications.

Turmeric, with its golden glow and healing touch, offers a natural remedy for inflammation, oxidative stress, and digestive woes. By harnessing the power of this ancient spice, we can nourish our bodies, soothe our souls, and embrace the vibrant tapestry of health and vitality. With turmeric as our ally, we embark on a journey of wellness, radiant with the promise of golden healing.

Boswellia: The Soothing Balm of Nature

Introduction

Boswellia, an ancient remedy with a storied past, emerges from the resin of the Boswellia serrata tree as a beacon of hope for those seeking relief from inflammation and joint discomfort. Revered for centuries in traditional medicine systems such as Ayurveda, boswellia offers a natural alternative to address a myriad of health concerns. In this chapter, we delve into the profound healing properties of boswellia and its role as a gentle yet powerful remedy for inflammation and joint health.

Understanding Boswellia

Botanical Background: Boswellia, also known as Indian frankincense, is a resinous extract derived from the Boswellia serrata tree, native to India, North Africa, and the Middle East. The resin, prized for its therapeutic properties, has been used for centuries in traditional medicine practices to alleviate pain, inflammation, and various ailments.

Medicinal Properties: Boswellia contains bioactive compounds known as boswellic acids, which possess anti-inflammatory, analgesic, and immunomodulatory effects. These compounds target key pathways involved in inflammation, making boswellia a valuable ally in managing chronic inflammatory conditions.

Harnessing the Power of Boswellia

Anti-inflammatory Action: Boswellia's primary claim to fame lies in its potent anti-inflammatory properties. Boswellic acids inhibit the activity of inflammatory enzymes such as 5-lipoxygenase (5-LOX), reducing the production of pro-inflammatory mediators and alleviating inflammation in the body.

Joint Health Support: Boswellia is particularly beneficial for promoting joint health and mobility. By reducing inflammation and inhibiting the breakdown of cartilage, boswellia helps to alleviate pain and stiffness associated with arthritis, osteoarthritis, and other inflammatory joint conditions.

Respiratory Wellness: Boswellia's anti-inflammatory and bronchodilator properties make it a valuable ally for respiratory health. It may help alleviate symptoms of asthma, bronchitis, and chronic obstructive pulmonary disease (COPD) by reducing inflammation in the airways and improving breathing.

How to Use Boswellia

Boswellia Supplements: Take boswellia supplements in capsule or tablet form for a convenient and concentrated dose of its therapeutic benefits. Look for standardized extracts containing a high percentage of boswellic acids for optimal efficacy.

Topical Applications: Apply boswellia oil or ointment topically to areas of inflammation or joint pain for localized relief. Boswellia-infused balms or creams can help soothe sore muscles, reduce swelling, and improve mobility.

Resin Incense: Burn boswellia resin as incense to purify the air and create a calming atmosphere. Boswellia resin has a rich, earthy aroma that promotes relaxation and spiritual well-being.

Safety Considerations

Boswellia is generally safe for most people when used as directed. However, individuals with certain medical conditions or those taking medications should consult with a healthcare professional before using boswellia supplements. Pregnant or breastfeeding women should also exercise caution when using boswellia.

Boswellia, with its ancient roots and modern-day applications, offers a natural solution for inflammation, joint pain, and respiratory wellness. By harnessing the power of boswellic acids, we can soothe inflammation, promote joint health, and enhance overall well-being. With boswellia as our ally, we embrace the healing gifts of nature and embark on a journey of vitality and resilience.

Willow Bark: Nature's Analgesic Ally

Introduction

Willow bark, with its ancient lineage and time-honored reputation, emerges from the depths of history as a natural remedy for pain and inflammation. Revered by ancient civilizations and cherished by herbalists throughout the ages, willow bark offers a gentle yet potent alternative to conventional pain relievers. In this chapter, we explore the remarkable properties of willow bark and its role as a soothing analgesic for various ailments.

Understanding Willow Bark

Botanical Background: Willow bark, derived from the bark of several species of willow trees, including Salix alba and Salix purpurea, has been used for centuries in traditional medicine for its pain-relieving and anti-inflammatory properties. The active compound responsible for its therapeutic effects is salicin, a natural precursor to aspirin.

Medicinal Properties: Willow bark contains salicin, a compound that acts as a natural pain reliever and anti-inflammatory agent. Salicin is converted to salicylic acid in the body, which exerts analgesic and anti-inflammatory effects similar to those of aspirin.

Harnessing the Power of Willow Bark

Pain Relief: Willow bark is primarily used to alleviate pain associated with various conditions, including headaches, menstrual cramps, muscle aches, and arthritis. Its analgesic properties help reduce pain sensations, making it a valuable alternative to conventional pain relievers for mild to moderate pain.

Anti-inflammatory Action: In addition to its pain-relieving effects, willow bark exhibits anti-inflammatory properties that can help reduce inflammation in the body. This makes it particularly beneficial for conditions characterized by inflammation, such as arthritis, tendonitis, and bursitis.

Fever Reduction: Willow bark's ability to lower fever has been recognized for centuries. By reducing fever, willow bark helps the body fight infection and promotes recovery from illness.

How to Use Willow Bark

Herbal Tea: Brew dried willow bark into a soothing herbal tea by steeping it in hot water for 10-15 minutes. Strain the tea and drink it warm or cold as needed for pain relief or fever reduction.

Tincture: Take willow bark tincture orally by diluting it in water or juice according to the manufacturer's instructions. Tinctures provide a concentrated dose of willow bark's active constituents for quick and effective pain relief.

Topical Applications: Apply willow bark-infused ointments or poultices topically to areas of pain or inflammation for localized relief. Willow bark creams or salves can help soothe sore muscles, reduce swelling, and promote healing.

Safety Considerations

While willow bark is generally considered safe for most people when used as directed, it may not be suitable for everyone. Individuals with allergies to aspirin or salicylates should avoid willow bark. Additionally, pregnant or breastfeeding women, as well as individuals taking blood-thinning medications or with certain medical conditions, should consult with a healthcare professional before using willow bark.

Willow bark, with its time-tested efficacy and gentle nature, offers a natural solution for pain relief, inflammation reduction, and fever reduction. By harnessing the power of salicin, we can soothe discomfort, promote healing, and enhance overall well-being. With willow bark as our ally, we embrace the ancient wisdom of herbal medicine and embark on a journey of holistic healing and vitality.

Devil's Claw: Nature's Soothing Remedy

Introduction

Devil's Claw, with its formidable name and remarkable properties, emerges from the African savanna as a potent herbal remedy for pain and inflammation. Revered by indigenous peoples for centuries, this claw-shaped fruit holds within it the promise of relief from various ailments. In this chapter, we explore the intriguing attributes of Devil's Claw and its role as a natural analgesic and anti-inflammatory agent.

Understanding Devil's Claw

Botanical Background: Devil's Claw, scientifically known as Harpagophytum procumbens, is a plant native to the Kalahari Desert regions of southern Africa. It derives its name from the distinctive hooks or "claws" that adorn its fruit, which inspired both awe and reverence among indigenous tribes who discovered its medicinal properties.

Medicinal Properties: Devil's Claw owes its therapeutic effects to its rich array of bioactive compounds, including iridoid glycosides, harpagoside, and harpagide. These compounds possess anti-inflammatory, analgesic, and antioxidant properties, making Devil's Claw a valuable ally in managing pain and inflammation.

Harnessing the Power of Devil's Claw

Pain Relief: Devil's Claw is primarily used to alleviate pain associated with various conditions, including arthritis, back pain, muscle aches, and headaches. Its analgesic properties help reduce pain sensations, providing relief for both acute and chronic pain.

Anti-inflammatory Action: In addition to its pain-relieving effects, Devil's Claw exhibits potent anti-inflammatory properties that can help reduce inflammation in the body. This makes it particularly beneficial for conditions characterized by inflammation, such as arthritis, tendonitis, and bursitis.

Digestive Support: Devil's Claw has been traditionally used to promote digestive health and alleviate gastrointestinal discomfort. It may help relieve symptoms of indigestion, bloating, and stomach ulcers by soothing inflammation in the digestive tract.

How to Use Devil's Claw

Herbal Tea: Brew dried Devil's Claw root into a soothing herbal tea by steeping it in hot water for 10-15 minutes. Strain the tea and drink it warm or cold as needed for pain relief or digestive support.

Capsules or Tablets: Take Devil's Claw supplements in capsule or tablet form for a convenient and concentrated dose of its therapeutic benefits. Follow the manufacturer's dosage recommendations for optimal results.

Topical Applications: Apply Devil's Claw-infused creams or ointments topically to areas of pain or inflammation for localized relief. Devil's Claw creams or salves can help soothe sore muscles, reduce swelling, and promote healing.

Safety Considerations

Devil's Claw is generally considered safe for most people when used as directed. However, it may not be suitable for everyone. Individuals with certain medical conditions, such as peptic ulcers or gallstones, should consult with a healthcare professional before using Devil's Claw. Pregnant or breastfeeding women should also exercise caution when using Devil's Claw.

Devil's Claw, with its unique shape and powerful properties, offers a natural solution for pain relief, inflammation reduction, and digestive support. By harnessing the power of its bioactive compounds, we can soothe discomfort, promote healing, and enhance overall well-being. With Devil's Claw as our ally, we embrace the healing wisdom of nature and embark on a journey of holistic wellness and vitality.

Herbal Approaches to Diabetes Management

Introduction

Diabetes, a chronic condition characterized by elevated blood sugar levels, poses significant challenges to millions worldwide. While conventional treatments such as insulin therapy and medication play a crucial role in managing diabetes, many individuals seek complementary approaches to support their health and well-being. In this chapter, we explore the role of herbal medicine in diabetes management, focusing on botanical allies that offer potential benefits for blood sugar control and overall health.

Understanding Diabetes

Types of Diabetes: Diabetes encompasses a spectrum of metabolic disorders, with the two main types being type 1 and type 2 diabetes. Type 1 diabetes is an autoimmune condition in which the body's immune system attacks and destroys insulin-producing cells in the pancreas. Type 2 diabetes, the more common form, occurs when the body becomes resistant to insulin or fails to produce enough insulin to maintain normal blood sugar levels.

Challenges of Diabetes Management: Managing diabetes involves maintaining blood sugar levels within a target range to prevent complications such as cardiovascular disease, kidney damage, nerve damage, and vision problems. Lifestyle modifications, including dietary changes, regular exercise, and medication, are essential components of diabetes management.

Herbal Approaches

Gymnema Sylvestre: Gymnema sylvestre, a plant native to India, has a long history of use in Ayurvedic medicine for its potential blood sugar-lowering effects. It may help improve insulin sensitivity, reduce sugar cravings, and lower blood sugar levels in individuals with type 2 diabetes.

Cinnamon: Cinnamon, a popular spice derived from the inner bark of trees belonging to the Cinnamomum genus, has been studied for its potential benefits in diabetes management. It may help improve insulin sensitivity, lower fasting blood sugar levels, and reduce postprandial blood sugar spikes.

Fenugreek: Fenugreek seeds, commonly used as a culinary spice in Indian cuisine, have been shown to have hypoglycemic effects. They may help lower blood sugar levels, improve insulin sensitivity, and reduce cholesterol levels in individuals with type 2 diabetes.

Bitter Melon: Bitter melon, also known as bitter gourd or Momordica charantia, is a tropical fruit that has been traditionally used in Asian and African medicine to lower blood sugar levels. It contains compounds that mimic insulin and may help improve glucose utilization in the body.

Incorporating Herbal Medicine

Consultation with Healthcare Provider: Before incorporating herbal remedies into your diabetes management plan, it is essential to consult with a healthcare provider, especially if you are taking medications or have underlying health conditions. Some herbs may interact with medications or have contraindications for certain individuals.

Integration with Conventional Treatment: Herbal medicine should complement, not replace, conventional diabetes treatments such as insulin therapy and medication. It can be used as part of a comprehensive approach to diabetes management, alongside dietary modifications, regular exercise, and monitoring of blood sugar levels.

Monitoring and Adjustment: Regular monitoring of blood sugar levels is crucial when using herbal remedies for diabetes management. Adjustments to dosage or treatment may be necessary based on individual response and changes in health status.

Herbal medicine offers a complementary approach to diabetes management, providing potential benefits for blood sugar control and overall health. By incorporating herbs such as gymnema sylvestre, cinnamon, fenugreek, and bitter melon into a comprehensive treatment plan, individuals with diabetes can optimize their health outcomes and improve their quality of life. With careful consideration, consultation with healthcare providers, and a holistic approach to wellness, herbal medicine can be a valuable ally in the journey towards better diabetes management and overall well-being.

Fenugreek: Nature's Blood Sugar Balancer

Introduction

Fenugreek, a humble herb with a powerhouse of health benefits, has long been revered in traditional medicine systems for its therapeutic properties. From culinary spice to herbal remedy, fenugreek holds a special place in the hearts and homes of many cultures worldwide. In this chapter, we delve into the extraordinary benefits of fenugreek and its role in promoting blood sugar balance and overall well-being.

Understanding Fenugreek

Botanical Background: Fenugreek (Trigonella foenum-graecum) is an annual herb native to the Mediterranean region, cultivated for its seeds and leaves, which are used in cooking and traditional medicine. The seeds, in particular, are prized for their unique flavor and medicinal properties.

Medicinal Properties: Fenugreek seeds are rich in bioactive compounds, including saponins, alkaloids, and fiber, which contribute to their therapeutic effects. Fenugreek is known for its potential to lower blood sugar levels, improve insulin sensitivity, and support digestive health.

Harnessing the Power of Fenugreek

Blood Sugar Regulation: Fenugreek seeds contain soluble fiber, which slows down the absorption of carbohydrates and sugars in the digestive tract, helping to stabilize blood sugar levels. Additionally, fenugreek may improve insulin sensitivity and reduce insulin resistance, making it beneficial for individuals with diabetes or prediabetes.

Cholesterol Management: Fenugreek seeds have been shown to reduce levels of LDL cholesterol (the "bad" cholesterol) and triglycerides, while increasing levels of HDL cholesterol (the "good" cholesterol). This may help improve cardiovascular health and reduce the risk of heart disease.

Digestive Support: Fenugreek seeds have a long history of use in traditional medicine for digestive complaints such as indigestion, bloating, and constipation. The soluble fiber in fenugreek seeds helps to bulk up stools and promote regular bowel movements, while the mucilage content soothes and protects the digestive tract.

How to Use Fenugreek

Herbal Tea: Brew fenugreek seeds into a soothing herbal tea by steeping them in hot water for 10-15 minutes. Strain the seeds and drink the tea warm or cold as needed to support blood sugar balance and digestive health.

Sprouted Seeds: Sprout fenugreek seeds by soaking them in water overnight and then draining and rinsing them several times a day until sprouts appear. Fenugreek sprouts can be added to salads, sandwiches, and wraps for a nutritious boost.

Supplements: Take fenugreek supplements in capsule or tablet form for a concentrated dose of its therapeutic benefits. Follow the manufacturer's dosage recommendations for optimal results.

Safety Considerations

Fenugreek is generally safe for most people when consumed in culinary amounts or taken as a supplement. However, high doses of fenugreek may cause gastrointestinal discomfort or allergic reactions in some individuals. Pregnant women should avoid fenugreek supplements, as they may stimulate uterine contractions.

Fenugreek, with its rich history and multifaceted benefits, offers a natural solution for blood sugar balance, cholesterol management, and digestive support. By harnessing the power of fenugreek seeds, we can optimize our health and well-being, one seed at a time. With fenugreek as our ally, we embrace the healing gifts of nature and embark on a journey towards vitality and resilience.

Bitter Melon: Nature's Blood Sugar Regulator

Introduction

Bitter melon, with its distinctive appearance and bitter taste, emerges as a potent healer in the realm of herbal medicine. Revered for centuries in traditional healing systems such as Ayurveda and Traditional Chinese Medicine (TCM), bitter melon offers a natural approach to managing blood sugar levels and supporting overall health. In this chapter, we explore the remarkable properties of bitter melon and its role in promoting blood sugar regulation and well-being.

Understanding Bitter Melon

Botanical Background: Bitter melon (Momordica charantia), also known as bitter gourd or karela, is a tropical vine belonging to the Cucurbitaceae family. Native to Asia, Africa, and the Caribbean, bitter melon is cultivated for its edible fruit, which has a distinctively bitter taste and is used in culinary dishes and traditional medicine.

Medicinal Properties: Bitter melon contains a variety of bioactive compounds, including charantin, vicine, and polypeptide-p, which contribute to its therapeutic effects. These compounds are believed to mimic the action of insulin and help regulate blood sugar levels in the body.

Harnessing the Power of Bitter Melon

Blood Sugar Regulation: Bitter melon is best known for its ability to lower blood sugar levels and improve glucose tolerance. It contains compounds that mimic insulin, helping to transport glucose from the bloodstream into cells for energy production. This can be particularly beneficial for individuals with diabetes or prediabetes.

Antioxidant Protection: Bitter melon is rich in antioxidants, including vitamins C and E, which help neutralize harmful free radicals and protect cells from oxidative damage. This antioxidant activity may help reduce inflammation, support immune function, and prevent chronic diseases associated with oxidative stress.

Digestive Health: Bitter melon has been traditionally used to promote digestive health and alleviate gastrointestinal discomfort. It contains enzymes that aid in the digestion of carbohydrates, fats, and proteins, as well as fiber that helps promote regular bowel movements and prevent constipation.

How to Use Bitter Melon

Culinary Delight: Incorporate bitter melon into your culinary repertoire by adding it to stir-fries, curries, soups, and salads. Its distinctive bitter flavor adds depth and complexity to dishes, while its therapeutic properties support overall health.

Juicing: Juice bitter melon along with other fruits and vegetables to create a refreshing and nutritious beverage. Bitter melon juice can be enjoyed on its own or mixed with other ingredients such as lemon, apple, or ginger for added flavor.

Supplements: Take bitter melon supplements in capsule or tablet form for a concentrated dose of its therapeutic benefits. Follow the manufacturer's dosage recommendations for optimal results.

Safety Considerations

Bitter melon is generally safe for most people when consumed in moderate amounts as part of a balanced diet. However, it may cause gastrointestinal upset or allergic reactions in some individuals, especially when consumed in large quantities or by those with certain medical conditions. Pregnant or breastfeeding women should avoid bitter melon due to its potential to stimulate uterine contractions.

Bitter melon, with its unique flavor and powerful healing properties, offers a natural approach to blood sugar regulation, antioxidant protection, and digestive health. By embracing the gifts of this remarkable fruit, we can optimize our health and well-being, one bitter bite at a time. With bitter melon as our ally, we embark on a journey of vitality, resilience, and holistic wellness.

Cinnamon: Nature's Sweet Spice with Healing Powers

Introduction

Cinnamon, with its warm aroma and distinctive flavor, has enchanted cultures for centuries as both a culinary delight and a potent healer. Beyond its role in adding depth and richness to dishes, cinnamon holds a wealth of therapeutic benefits that have been treasured in traditional medicine systems worldwide. In this chapter, we explore the extraordinary properties of cinnamon and its profound impact on health and well-being.

Understanding Cinnamon

Botanical Background: Cinnamon is obtained from the inner bark of trees belonging to the genus Cinnamomum, native to Sri Lanka, India, and Southeast Asia. There are several varieties of cinnamon, with Ceylon cinnamon (Cinnamomum verum) and Cassia cinnamon (Cinnamomum cassia) being the most commonly used for their culinary and medicinal properties.

Medicinal Properties: Cinnamon owes its therapeutic effects to its rich array of bioactive compounds, including cinnamaldehyde, cinnamic acid, and cinnamate. These compounds possess antioxidant, anti-inflammatory, antimicrobial, and blood sugar-regulating properties, making cinnamon a versatile ally in promoting health and wellness.

Harnessing the Power of Cinnamon

Blood Sugar Regulation: Cinnamon is renowned for its ability to improve blood sugar control and insulin sensitivity, making it particularly beneficial for individuals with diabetes or prediabetes. It helps lower fasting blood sugar levels, reduce insulin resistance, and improve glucose metabolism, leading to better overall glycemic control.

Antioxidant Protection: Cinnamon is rich in antioxidants, which help neutralize harmful free radicals and protect cells from oxidative damage. This antioxidant activity may help reduce inflammation, support immune function, and lower the risk of chronic diseases such as heart disease, cancer, and neurodegenerative disorders.

Anti-inflammatory Effects: Cinnamon contains compounds that inhibit inflammatory pathways in the body, helping to reduce inflammation and alleviate symptoms of inflammatory conditions such as arthritis, asthma, and inflammatory bowel disease (IBD).

How to Use Cinnamon

Culinary Delight: Incorporate cinnamon into your culinary creations by adding it to baked goods, oatmeal, yogurt, smoothies, and savory dishes such as curries and stews. Its warm and spicy flavor adds depth and complexity to a wide range of dishes, making it a versatile and delicious spice.

Cinnamon Tea: Brew cinnamon sticks or ground cinnamon into a soothing herbal tea by steeping them in hot water for 10-15 minutes. Strain the tea and enjoy it warm or cold as a comforting beverage with potential health benefits.

Supplements: Take cinnamon supplements in capsule or tablet form for a concentrated dose of its therapeutic benefits. Look for supplements that contain Ceylon cinnamon for optimal potency and efficacy.

Safety Considerations

Cinnamon is generally safe for most people when consumed in culinary amounts or taken as a supplement. However, high doses of cinnamon may cause gastrointestinal upset or allergic reactions in some individuals. Pregnant women should avoid taking cinnamon supplements, as they may stimulate uterine contractions.

Cinnamon, with its sweet aroma and healing touch, offers a natural solution for blood sugar regulation, antioxidant protection, and inflammation reduction. By embracing the gifts of this remarkable spice, we can enhance our health and well-being, one sprinkle at a time. With cinnamon as our ally, we embark on a journey of vitality, flavor, and holistic wellness.

Gymnema: The Sugar Destroyer

Introduction

Gymnema, with its ancient roots in Ayurvedic medicine, emerges as a powerful ally in the battle against sugar cravings and blood sugar imbalances. Known as the "sugar destroyer," this remarkable herb has been treasured for centuries for its unique ability to support healthy glucose metabolism and promote overall well-being. In this chapter, we delve into the extraordinary properties of gymnema and its role in sugar regulation and health.

Understanding Gymnema

Botanical Background: Gymnema (Gymnema sylvestre) is a woody climbing vine native to the tropical forests of India, Africa, and Australia. Its leaves, when chewed, exhibit a remarkable property: the ability to temporarily suppress the taste of sweetness. This unique characteristic has earned gymnema its reputation as the "sugar destroyer" in traditional medicine.

Medicinal Properties: Gymnema owes its therapeutic effects to its bioactive compounds, including gymnemic acids and gymnemasaponins. These compounds are believed to block sugar receptors on the taste buds, reduce sugar absorption in the intestines, and enhance insulin production and sensitivity, leading to better blood sugar control.

Harnessing the Power of Gymnema

Sugar Craving Management: Gymnema is renowned for its ability to reduce sugar cravings and support weight management efforts. By blocking the taste of sweetness on the tongue, gymnema can help curb the desire for sugary foods and beverages, making it easier to adhere to a healthy diet and lifestyle.

Blood Sugar Regulation: Gymnema helps regulate blood sugar levels by enhancing insulin secretion and sensitivity, improving glucose uptake by cells, and reducing glucose absorption in the intestines. This makes it beneficial for individuals with diabetes or prediabetes who are seeking natural ways to manage their condition.

Cholesterol and Lipid Control: Gymnema has been shown to have lipid-lowering effects, helping to reduce levels of LDL cholesterol (the "bad" cholesterol) and triglycerides, while increasing levels of HDL cholesterol (the "good" cholesterol). This may contribute to improved cardiovascular health and reduced risk of heart disease.

How to Use Gymnema

Herbal Tea: Brew dried gymnema leaves into a soothing herbal tea by steeping them in hot water for 10-15 minutes. Strain the tea and drink it warm or cold as needed to support blood sugar regulation and reduce sugar cravings.

Supplements: Take gymnema supplements in capsule or tablet form for a concentrated dose of its therapeutic benefits. Look for supplements that contain standardized extracts of gymnema for optimal potency and efficacy.

Chewing Leaves: Chew fresh gymnema leaves or dried leaf powder before meals to temporarily suppress the taste of sweetness and reduce sugar cravings.

Safety Considerations

Gymnema is generally safe for most people when consumed in moderate amounts. However, pregnant or breastfeeding women, as well as individuals taking medications for diabetes or blood sugar management, should consult with a healthcare professional before using gymnema supplements.

Gymnema, with its unique ability to curb sugar cravings and support blood sugar regulation, offers a natural solution for individuals seeking to improve their health and well-being. By harnessing the power of this remarkable herb, we can overcome the allure of sugar, balance our blood sugar levels, and embark on a journey of vitality and resilience. With gymnema as our ally, we embrace the sweetness of life without succumbing to its pitfalls, and we stride confidently towards a healthier future.

Herbal Support for Cardiovascular Health

Introduction

Cardiovascular health is paramount to overall well-being, as the heart and blood vessels play a vital role in delivering oxygen and nutrients to every cell in the body. While lifestyle factors such as diet, exercise, and stress management are crucial for maintaining heart health, herbal medicine offers a complementary approach to support cardiovascular function and reduce the risk of heart disease. In this chapter, we explore the role of herbal remedies in promoting cardiovascular health and reducing the risk of cardiovascular disease.

Understanding Cardiovascular Health

The Importance of Cardiovascular Health: The cardiovascular system, comprising the heart and blood vessels, is responsible for circulating blood throughout the body, delivering oxygen and nutrients to tissues and organs, and removing waste products. Maintaining cardiovascular health is essential for preventing conditions such as heart disease, stroke, and hypertension.

Risk Factors for Cardiovascular Disease: Several factors contribute to the development of cardiovascular disease, including high blood pressure, high cholesterol levels, diabetes, obesity, smoking, sedentary lifestyle, and stress. Addressing these risk factors through lifestyle modifications and herbal interventions can help reduce the risk of heart disease and improve overall cardiovascular health.

Herbal Support for Cardiovascular Health

Hawthorn: Hawthorn (Crataegus spp.) is a renowned herb for heart health, traditionally used to support cardiovascular function and reduce the risk of heart disease. It contains compounds that help dilate blood vessels, improve blood flow, regulate blood pressure, and strengthen the heart muscle.

Garlic: Garlic (Allium sativum) has long been prized for its cardiovascular benefits, including its ability to lower blood pressure, reduce cholesterol levels, prevent blood clot formation, and improve circulation. It contains sulfur compounds that have vasodilatory and anti-inflammatory effects, promoting heart health.

Ginkgo Biloba: Ginkgo biloba is an ancient herb with modern-day applications in cardiovascular health. It improves circulation, enhances blood flow to the brain and extremities, reduces inflammation, and acts as an antioxidant, protecting blood vessels from damage.

Turmeric: Turmeric (Curcuma longa) is renowned for its anti-inflammatory and antioxidant properties, which make it beneficial for cardiovascular health. It helps reduce inflammation in blood vessels, lower cholesterol levels, prevent blood clot formation, and improve endothelial function.

Incorporating Herbal Medicine

Consultation with Healthcare Provider: Before incorporating herbal remedies into your cardiovascular health regimen, it is essential to consult with a healthcare provider, especially if you are taking medications or have underlying health conditions. Some herbs may interact with medications or have contraindications for certain individuals.

Integration with Lifestyle Modifications: Herbal medicine should complement, not replace, lifestyle modifications such as a heart-healthy diet, regular exercise, smoking cessation, stress management, and weight management. By integrating herbal remedies with these lifestyle changes, you can optimize your cardiovascular health and reduce the risk of heart disease.

Monitoring and Adjustment: Regular monitoring of cardiovascular risk factors such as blood pressure, cholesterol levels, and blood sugar levels is crucial when using herbal remedies for cardiovascular health. Adjustments to dosage or treatment may be necessary based on individual response and changes in health status.

Herbal medicine offers a valuable adjunct to lifestyle modifications in promoting cardiovascular health and reducing the risk of heart disease. By harnessing the power of herbs such as hawthorn, garlic, ginkgo biloba, and turmeric, individuals can support healthy circulation, reduce inflammation, and protect their hearts against disease. With a holistic approach that combines herbal interventions with healthy lifestyle choices, we can nurture our cardiovascular health and embark on a journey of vitality and longevity.

Hawthorn: Nature's Heart Tonic

Introduction

Hawthorn, with its delicate blossoms and vibrant berries, stands as a symbol of vitality and resilience in the world of herbal medicine. Revered for centuries for its cardiovascular benefits, hawthorn offers a natural approach to supporting heart health and promoting overall well-being. In this chapter, we delve into the remarkable properties of hawthorn and its role as a heart tonic and cardiovascular ally.

Understanding Hawthorn

Botanical Background: Hawthorn (Crataegus spp.) is a thorny shrub or small tree belonging to the rose family (Rosaceae), native to temperate regions of Europe, Asia, and North America. It is characterized by its clusters of white or pink flowers, followed by bright red berries, which are rich in bioactive compounds with medicinal properties.

Medicinal Properties: Hawthorn is prized for its cardiovascular benefits, attributed to its rich array of bioactive compounds, including flavonoids, oligomeric proanthocyanidins (OPCs), and triterpenoids. These compounds exert a range of effects on the cardiovascular system, including vasodilation, antioxidant activity, and support for cardiac function.

Harnessing the Power of Hawthorn

Heart Health Support: Hawthorn is renowned for its ability to support heart health and reduce the risk of cardiovascular disease. It helps dilate blood vessels, improve blood flow, regulate blood pressure, and strengthen the heart muscle, making it beneficial for individuals with conditions such as hypertension, angina, and heart failure.

Antioxidant Protection: Hawthorn berries are rich in antioxidants, which help neutralize harmful free radicals and protect cells from oxidative damage. This antioxidant activity may help reduce inflammation, prevent plaque buildup in the arteries, and lower the risk of atherosclerosis and heart disease.

Stress Reduction: Hawthorn has mild sedative properties that can help reduce stress and anxiety, which are risk factors for heart disease. By promoting relaxation and calming the nervous system, hawthorn may indirectly support cardiovascular health and reduce the risk of stress-related heart problems.

How to Use Hawthorn

Herbal Tea: Brew dried hawthorn berries or leaves into a soothing herbal tea by steeping them in hot water for 10-15 minutes. Strain the tea and drink it warm or cold as needed to support heart health and promote relaxation.

Tincture or Extract: Take hawthorn tincture or liquid extract orally, following the manufacturer's dosage recommendations. Tinctures provide a concentrated dose of hawthorn's therapeutic compounds and can be easily added to water or juice for convenient consumption.

Capsules or Tablets: Take hawthorn supplements in capsule or tablet form for a convenient and standardized dose of its cardiovascular benefits. Follow the manufacturer's dosage recommendations for optimal results.

Safety Considerations

Hawthorn is generally safe for most people when consumed in moderate amounts. However, pregnant or breastfeeding women, as well as individuals taking medications for heart conditions or blood pressure, should consult with a healthcare professional before using hawthorn supplements.

Hawthorn, with its time-honored reputation as a heart tonic and cardiovascular ally, offers a natural approach to supporting heart health and promoting overall well-being. By harnessing the power of hawthorn's bioactive compounds, we can nourish our hearts, protect our blood vessels, and embrace a life of vitality and resilience. With hawthorn as our ally, we stride confidently towards a future of cardiovascular wellness and longevity.

Garlic: Nature's Heart Protector

Introduction

Garlic, with its pungent aroma and distinctive flavor, has been revered for centuries as a culinary staple and a potent healer in traditional medicine systems worldwide. Beyond its culinary uses, garlic holds a wealth of therapeutic benefits, particularly for cardiovascular health. In this chapter, we explore the remarkable properties of garlic and its role as a heart protector and overall health ally.

Understanding Garlic

Botanical Background: Garlic (Allium sativum) is a member of the onion family (Alliaceae) and is native to Central Asia. It has been cultivated for thousands of years for its culinary and medicinal properties. Garlic bulbs consist of multiple cloves enclosed in a papery sheath, each containing sulfur compounds that contribute to its unique aroma and health benefits.

Medicinal Properties: Garlic owes its therapeutic effects to its rich array of bioactive compounds, including allicin, diallyl sulfide, and S-allyl cysteine. These sulfur-containing compounds have antioxidant, anti-inflammatory, antimicrobial, and cardiovascular-protective properties, making garlic a versatile remedy for various health conditions.

Harnessing the Power of Garlic

Heart Health Support: Garlic is renowned for its cardiovascular benefits, including its ability to lower blood pressure, reduce cholesterol levels, prevent blood clot formation, and improve circulation. Its sulfur compounds help relax blood vessels, reduce inflammation in the arteries, and protect against atherosclerosis and heart disease.

Antioxidant Protection: Garlic is rich in antioxidants, which help neutralize harmful free radicals and protect cells from oxidative damage. This antioxidant activity may help reduce inflammation, prevent plaque buildup in the arteries, and lower the risk of cardiovascular disease, including heart attacks and strokes.

Immune System Enhancement: Garlic has immune-boosting properties that can help defend the body against infections and illnesses. Its sulfur compounds have antimicrobial and antiviral effects, making garlic beneficial for preventing and treating colds, flu, and other respiratory infections.

How to Use Garlic

Raw Garlic: Consume raw garlic cloves for maximum health benefits. Crush or mince fresh garlic cloves and let them sit for a few minutes to activate the allicin content before consuming them. You can eat raw garlic on its own or add it to salads, dressings, dips, or spreads.

Cooked Garlic: Incorporate cooked garlic into your meals by sautéing, roasting, or baking it with vegetables, meats, grains, or legumes. Cooking garlic reduces its pungency while preserving its health-promoting properties, making it a versatile and flavorful addition to various dishes.

Garlic Supplements: Take garlic supplements in capsule or tablet form for a concentrated dose of its therapeutic benefits. Look for supplements that contain standardized extracts of garlic for optimal potency and efficacy. Follow the manufacturer's dosage recommendations for best results.

Safety Considerations

Garlic is generally safe for most people when consumed in culinary amounts or taken as a supplement. However, high doses of garlic may cause gastrointestinal upset or allergic reactions in some individuals. Pregnant or breastfeeding women, as well as individuals taking blood-thinning medications, should consult with a healthcare professional before using garlic supplements.

Garlic, with its potent aroma and profound healing properties, stands as a stalwart defender of heart health and overall well-being. By embracing the gifts of this remarkable bulb, we can nourish our bodies, protect our hearts, and thrive in a life of vitality and resilience. With garlic as our ally, we stride confidently towards a future of cardiovascular wellness and longevity.

Hibiscus: The Heart's Floral Ally

Introduction

Hibiscus, with its vibrant blooms and refreshing tang, emerges not only as a sight to behold but also as a potent healer in the realm of herbal medicine. Revered for centuries in cultures around the world, hibiscus offers a natural approach to supporting cardiovascular health and promoting overall well-being. In this chapter, we explore the remarkable properties of hibiscus and its role as a floral ally for the heart.

Understanding Hibiscus

Botanical Background: Hibiscus, belonging to the genus Hibiscus and the Malvaceae family, encompasses hundreds of species of flowering plants native to tropical and subtropical regions. Known for its large, colorful flowers, hibiscus has been cultivated for its ornamental beauty as well as its culinary and medicinal uses.

Medicinal Properties: Hibiscus flowers, particularly those of Hibiscus sabdariffa, are prized for their medicinal properties, including antioxidant, anti-inflammatory, and cardiovascular-protective effects. Hibiscus contains bioactive compounds such as flavonoids, anthocyanins, and polyphenols, which contribute to its therapeutic benefits.

Harnessing the Power of Hibiscus

Heart Health Support: Hibiscus is renowned for its cardiovascular benefits, particularly its ability to lower blood pressure and improve lipid profiles. Studies have shown that hibiscus tea consumption may help reduce both systolic and diastolic blood pressure levels, making it beneficial for individuals with hypertension or prehypertension.

Antioxidant Protection: Hibiscus is rich in antioxidants, which help neutralize harmful free radicals and protect cells from oxidative damage. This antioxidant activity may help reduce inflammation, prevent plaque buildup in the arteries, and lower the risk of cardiovascular disease, including heart attacks and strokes.

Kidney Health: Hibiscus has diuretic properties that can help promote kidney health by increasing urine output and flushing out toxins and waste products from the body. By supporting kidney function, hibiscus may indirectly benefit cardiovascular health and reduce the risk of conditions such as kidney stones and urinary tract infections.

How to Use Hibiscus

Herbal Tea: Brew dried hibiscus flowers into a refreshing herbal tea by steeping them in hot water for 5-10 minutes. Strain the tea and drink it warm or cold as a delicious and healthful beverage. You can enjoy hibiscus tea on its own or mix it with other herbs or flavorings for added variety.

Infusions: Infuse hibiscus flowers in cold water to create a refreshing herbal infusion. Simply place dried hibiscus flowers in a container with cold water and let steep for several hours or overnight in the refrigerator. Strain and enjoy the infused water for a hydrating and antioxidant-rich beverage.

Tinctures: Take hibiscus tinctures orally, following the manufacturer's dosage recommendations. Tinctures provide a concentrated dose of hibiscus's therapeutic compounds and can be easily added to water or juice for convenient consumption.

Safety Considerations

Hibiscus is generally safe for most people when consumed in moderate amounts. However, high doses of hibiscus may cause gastrointestinal upset or allergic reactions in some individuals. Pregnant or breastfeeding women, as well as individuals taking medications for blood pressure or other cardiovascular conditions, should consult with a healthcare professional before using hibiscus supplements.

Hibiscus, with its radiant beauty and healing touch, offers a natural approach to supporting cardiovascular health and promoting overall well-being. By harnessing the power of hibiscus's bioactive compounds, we can nurture our hearts, protect our blood vessels, and embrace a life of vitality and resilience. With hibiscus as our floral ally, we stride confidently towards a future of cardiovascular wellness and longevity.

Green Tea: The Elixir of Vitality

Introduction

Green tea, celebrated for its delicate flavor and potent health benefits, has been cherished for centuries in Asian cultures as a symbol of vitality and longevity. Renowned for its rich antioxidant content and numerous therapeutic properties, green tea offers a natural approach to promoting overall well-being, including cardiovascular health, weight management, and cognitive function. In this chapter, we explore the extraordinary properties of green tea and its role as an elixir of vitality.

Understanding Green Tea

Botanical Background: Green tea, derived from the leaves of the Camellia sinensis plant, is a type of tea that undergoes minimal oxidation during processing, preserving its natural color and flavor. Originating in China thousands of years ago, green tea has since spread throughout Asia and the world, becoming a beloved beverage and a cornerstone of traditional medicine.

Medicinal Properties: Green tea owes its health-promoting effects to its rich array of bioactive compounds, including catechins, flavonoids, and polyphenols. These antioxidants have anti-inflammatory, antimicrobial, and cardiovascular-protective properties, making green tea a powerful ally for health and wellness.

Harnessing the Power of Green Tea

Heart Health Support: Green tea is renowned for its cardiovascular benefits, including its ability to lower blood pressure, reduce cholesterol levels, and improve endothelial function. The catechins in green tea help relax blood vessels, inhibit cholesterol absorption, and prevent the formation of blood clots, reducing the risk of heart disease and stroke.

Weight Management: Green tea has been shown to promote weight loss and fat burning, making it a popular supplement for individuals looking to manage their weight. The catechins and caffeine in green tea help boost metabolism, increase fat oxidation, and suppress appetite, leading to greater calorie expenditure and fat loss.

Brain Health: Green tea contains compounds that support cognitive function and may help protect against age-related cognitive decline and neurodegenerative diseases such as Alzheimer's and Parkinson's. The antioxidants in green tea help reduce oxidative stress, inflammation, and damage to brain cells, promoting brain health and longevity.

How to Enjoy Green Tea

Brewed Tea: Brew green tea leaves in hot water for 2-3 minutes to extract their flavor and therapeutic compounds. Strain the tea and enjoy it plain or with a slice of lemon or a drizzle of honey for added flavor. Green tea can be enjoyed hot or cold, depending on personal preference.

Matcha: Enjoy the vibrant green color and concentrated flavor of matcha, a powdered form of green tea made from finely ground tea leaves. Whisk matcha powder with hot water to create a frothy and invigorating beverage that can be enjoyed on its own or incorporated into recipes such as smoothies, lattes, and desserts.

Supplements: Take green tea supplements in capsule or tablet form for a concentrated dose of its therapeutic benefits. Look for supplements that contain standardized extracts of green tea for optimal potency and efficacy. Follow the manufacturer's dosage recommendations for best results.

Safety Considerations

While green tea is generally safe for most people when consumed in moderate amounts, excessive intake of green tea or green tea supplements may cause side effects such as insomnia, anxiety, digestive upset, or liver damage in sensitive individuals. Pregnant or breastfeeding women, as well as individuals taking medications or with underlying health conditions, should consult with a healthcare professional before using green tea supplements.

Green tea, with its refreshing flavor and myriad health benefits, stands as a beacon of vitality and longevity in the realm of herbal medicine. By embracing the gifts of green tea's antioxidants and bioactive compounds, we can nourish our bodies, protect our hearts and brains, and enhance our overall well-being. With green tea as our elixir of vitality, we embark on a journey of health, vitality, and longevity, one sip at a time.

Nurturing Mental Health and Emotional Well-being: The Herbal Approach

Introduction

In the fast-paced modern world, maintaining mental health and emotional well-being is essential for overall wellness and quality of life. While various factors contribute to mental health, including genetics, environment, and life experiences, herbal medicine offers a holistic approach to support mental clarity, emotional balance, and resilience. In this chapter, we explore the therapeutic potential of herbs in nurturing mental health and emotional well-being.

Understanding Mental Health and Emotional Well-being

The Importance of Mental Health: Mental health encompasses emotional, psychological, and social well-being, influencing how individuals think, feel, and act. It affects every aspect of life, from relationships and work performance to physical health and quality of life. Mental health is not merely the absence of mental illness but also the presence of positive attributes such as resilience, self-esteem, and emotional intelligence.

Factors Affecting Mental Health: Mental health is influenced by a complex interplay of biological, psychological, and social factors. Genetics, brain chemistry, traumatic experiences, stress, lifestyle habits, and social support networks all contribute to mental health outcomes. Cultivating resilience, coping skills, and healthy habits can help individuals navigate life's challenges and maintain emotional well-being.

Herbal Support for Mental Health and Emotional Well-being

Adaptogens: Adaptogenic herbs such as ashwagandha, rhodiola, and holy basil help the body adapt to stress and promote resilience. They modulate the body's stress response system, regulate cortisol levels, and support adrenal gland function, helping individuals cope with stress more effectively and maintain emotional balance.

Nervines: Nervine herbs such as chamomile, lemon balm, and passionflower have calming and soothing effects on the nervous system. They help reduce anxiety, promote relaxation, and improve sleep quality, making them valuable allies for managing stress, anxiety, and insomnia.

Mood Lifters: Certain herbs such as St. John's wort, saffron, and lemon verbena have mood-lifting properties that can help alleviate symptoms of depression and enhance emotional well-being. They work by modulating neurotransmitter levels, increasing serotonin and dopamine levels, and promoting a positive outlook on life.

Incorporating Herbal Medicine into Daily Life

Herbal Teas: Brew herbal teas using dried herbs or tea bags for a soothing and therapeutic beverage. Enjoy a cup of chamomile tea before bed to promote relaxation and improve sleep quality, or sip on a blend of lemon balm and lavender tea to ease anxiety and stress.

Tinctures and Extracts: Take herbal tinctures or liquid extracts orally for a convenient and concentrated dose of therapeutic herbs. Add a few drops of ashwagandha tincture to your morning smoothie for stress relief and energy support, or use passionflower extract to calm the mind and promote relaxation during times of tension.

Aromatherapy: Use essential oils derived from aromatic herbs such as lavender, bergamot, and frankincense for aromatherapy. Diffuse essential oils in your home or workplace to create a calming and uplifting atmosphere, or add a few drops to a warm bath for a relaxing and rejuvenating experience.

Safety Considerations

While herbs are generally safe when used appropriately, it's essential to consult with a qualified healthcare practitioner before using herbal remedies, especially if you are pregnant, breastfeeding, or taking medications. Some herbs may interact with medications or have contraindications for certain individuals, so it's crucial to seek personalized guidance to ensure safe and effective use.

Herbal medicine offers a holistic approach to nurturing mental health and emotional well-being, providing valuable support for stress management, anxiety relief, and mood enhancement. By incorporating adaptogens, nervines, and mood lifters into daily life, individuals can cultivate resilience, emotional balance, and inner peace. With herbal medicine as a gentle and effective ally, we embark on a journey of self-care, self-discovery, and holistic wellness, honoring the interconnectedness of mind, body, and spirit.

Finding Calm in the Storm: Herbal Solutions for Anxiety and Stress Relief

Introduction

In today's fast-paced world, feelings of anxiety and stress have become increasingly common, affecting millions of individuals worldwide. While stress is a natural response to challenging situations, chronic stress and anxiety can take a toll on mental and emotional well-being, impacting daily functioning and quality of life. In this chapter, we explore the therapeutic potential of herbs in providing relief from anxiety and stress, promoting relaxation, and restoring inner calm.

Understanding Anxiety and Stress

The Nature of Anxiety: Anxiety is a natural response to perceived threats or challenges, activating the body's fight-or-flight response and preparing it to deal with danger. However, when anxiety becomes excessive or chronic, it can interfere with daily life, leading to feelings of unease, apprehension, and fear that persist even in the absence of real danger.

The Impact of Stress: Stress is the body's physiological and psychological response to external pressures or demands, triggering a cascade of hormonal and physiological changes designed to help cope with perceived threats. While acute stress can be beneficial in certain situations, chronic stress can have detrimental effects on physical, mental, and emotional health.

Herbal Support for Anxiety and Stress Relief

Adaptogens: Adaptogenic herbs such as ashwagandha, rhodiola, and holy basil help the body adapt to stress and promote resilience. They modulate the body's stress response system, regulate cortisol levels, and support adrenal gland function, helping individuals cope with stress more effectively and maintain emotional balance.

Nervines: Nervine herbs such as chamomile, lemon balm, and passionflower have calming and soothing effects on the nervous system. They help reduce anxiety, promote relaxation, and improve sleep quality, making them valuable allies for managing stress and anxiety.

Aromatic Herbs: Aromatic herbs such as lavender, bergamot, and frankincense have calming and uplifting properties that can help alleviate anxiety and promote emotional well-being. They can be used in aromatherapy, massage oils, or herbal baths to induce relaxation and reduce tension.

Incorporating Herbal Remedies into Daily Life

Herbal Teas: Brew herbal teas using dried herbs or tea bags for a soothing and therapeutic beverage. Enjoy a cup of chamomile tea before bed to promote relaxation and improve sleep quality, or sip on a blend of lemon balm and passionflower tea during the day to ease anxiety and stress.

Tinctures and Extracts: Take herbal tinctures or liquid extracts orally for a convenient and concentrated dose of therapeutic herbs. Add a few drops of ashwagandha tincture to your morning smoothie for stress relief and energy support, or use lavender extract to calm the mind and promote relaxation during times of tension.

Aromatherapy: Use essential oils derived from aromatic herbs such as lavender, bergamot, and frankincense for aromatherapy. Diffuse essential oils in your home or workplace to create a calming and uplifting atmosphere, or add a few drops to a warm bath for a relaxing and rejuvenating experience.

Safety Considerations

While herbs are generally safe when used appropriately, it's essential to consult with a qualified healthcare practitioner before using herbal remedies, especially if you are pregnant, breastfeeding, or taking medications. Some herbs may interact with medications or have contraindications for certain individuals, so it's crucial to seek personalized guidance to ensure safe and effective use.

Herbal medicine offers a gentle and effective approach to relieving anxiety and stress, promoting relaxation, and restoring inner calm. By incorporating adaptogens, nervines, and aromatic herbs into daily life, individuals can cultivate resilience, emotional balance, and peace of mind. With herbal remedies as allies in the journey toward mental and emotional well-being, we can find solace in the midst of life's challenges and embrace a life of tranquility and serenity.

Ashwagandha: The Herb of Resilience

Introduction

Ashwagandha, revered for centuries in Ayurvedic medicine as a potent adaptogen, emerges as a beacon of resilience and vitality in the world of herbal medicine. With its robust roots and rejuvenating properties, ashwagandha offers a natural approach to promoting overall well-being and enhancing resilience to stress. In this chapter, we explore the remarkable properties of ashwagandha and its role as an herb of resilience.

Understanding Ashwagandha

Botanical Background: Ashwagandha (Withania somnifera), also known as Indian ginseng or winter cherry, is a small shrub native to the dry regions of India, the Middle East, and North Africa. Its name, which translates to "smell of horse" in Sanskrit, alludes to its distinct odor and traditional use as a strength-enhancing herb.

Medicinal Properties: Ashwagandha is prized for its adaptogenic properties, meaning it helps the body adapt to stress and maintain balance in the face of external challenges. It contains bioactive compounds such as withanolides, alkaloids, and steroidal lactones, which contribute to its therapeutic effects on the nervous, immune, and endocrine systems.

Harnessing the Power of Ashwagandha

Stress Reduction: Ashwagandha is renowned for its ability to reduce stress and promote relaxation. It helps regulate cortisol levels, the body's primary stress hormone, and modulate the body's stress response system, leading to a sense of calm and emotional stability even in the face of challenging situations.

Energy and Vitality: Ashwagandha has invigorating properties that help boost energy levels and enhance overall vitality. By supporting adrenal gland function and improving mitochondrial health, ashwagandha increases cellular energy production, reduces fatigue, and enhances physical and mental stamina.

Immune System Support: Ashwagandha has immunomodulatory effects that help regulate immune function and enhance resistance to infections and illnesses. It stimulates the production of white blood cells, antibodies, and other immune factors, strengthening the body's defenses and promoting optimal immune health.

How to Use Ashwagandha

Powder: Take ashwagandha powder orally by mixing it with water, juice, milk, or smoothies. Start with a small dose and gradually increase as needed to achieve the desired effect. Ashwagandha powder can also be added to recipes such as soups, stews, and baked goods for an extra boost of vitality.

Capsules or Tablets: Take ashwagandha supplements in capsule or tablet form for a convenient and standardized dose of its therapeutic benefits. Look for supplements that contain standardized extracts of ashwagandha for optimal potency and efficacy. Follow the manufacturer's dosage recommendations for best results.

Tinctures: Take ashwagandha tinctures orally by diluting them in water or juice and consuming them as directed. Tinctures provide a concentrated dose of ashwagandha's bioactive compounds and are easily absorbed by the body for quick and effective results.

Safety Considerations

Ashwagandha is generally safe for most people when consumed in moderate amounts. However, pregnant or breastfeeding women, as well as individuals with underlying health conditions or taking medications, should consult with a healthcare professional before using ashwagandha supplements. Some people may experience mild side effects such as gastrointestinal upset or drowsiness, especially when taking high doses of ashwagandha.

Ashwagandha, with its adaptogenic properties and rejuvenating effects, offers a natural approach to promoting resilience, reducing stress, and enhancing vitality. By harnessing the power of this remarkable herb, individuals can navigate life's challenges with greater ease, maintain emotional balance, and cultivate a sense of well-being from within. With ashwagandha as an ally in the journey toward resilience and vitality, we embrace life's ups and downs with grace and fortitude, embodying the spirit of resilience in mind, body, and spirit.

Valerian: Nature's Calming Remedy

Introduction

Valerian, with its delicate flowers and earthy fragrance, emerges as a gentle yet powerful ally in the quest for relaxation and tranquility. For centuries, this herb has been cherished for its calming properties, offering a natural solution for promoting restful sleep and easing nervous tension. In this chapter, we explore the remarkable properties of valerian and its role as nature's calming remedy.

Understanding Valerian

Botanical Background: Valerian (Valeriana officinalis) is a perennial flowering plant native to Europe and Asia, although it now grows in various parts of the world with temperate climates. The plant features clusters of small, fragrant white or pink flowers and deeply lobed leaves. Valerian root, the part of the plant used medicinally, contains a complex mixture of compounds that contribute to its therapeutic effects.

Medicinal Properties: Valerian is prized for its sedative, anxiolytic, and hypnotic properties, making it a popular remedy for promoting relaxation, easing nervousness, and improving sleep quality. Its primary bioactive compounds include valerenic acid, valepotriates, and volatile oils, which exert calming effects on the nervous system.

Harnessing the Power of Valerian

Sleep Support: Valerian is best known for its ability to promote restful sleep and alleviate insomnia. It helps reduce the time it takes to fall asleep, improve sleep quality, and enhance overall sleep duration, making it an effective alternative to conventional sleep aids. Valerian works by increasing levels of gamma-aminobutyric acid (GABA), a neurotransmitter that promotes relaxation and regulates sleep-wake cycles.

Anxiety Relief: Valerian has anxiolytic properties that help reduce feelings of nervousness, tension, and anxiety. It modulates neurotransmitter activity in the brain, including serotonin and norepinephrine, which play key roles in mood regulation and emotional well-being. Valerian's calming effects can help soothe frazzled nerves and promote a sense of inner peace.

Muscle Relaxation: Valerian has muscle-relaxant properties that can help ease tension and stiffness in the body. It may be beneficial for individuals experiencing muscle spasms, cramps, or discomfort associated with stress or physical exertion. Valerian's calming effects extend beyond the mind to the muscles, promoting overall relaxation and comfort.

How to Use Valerian

Herbal Tea: Brew valerian root into a soothing herbal tea by steeping it in hot water for 5-10 minutes. Strain the tea and drink it before bedtime to promote relaxation and improve sleep quality. You can also combine valerian with other calming herbs such as chamomile or lemon balm for added flavor and benefits.

Tinctures and Extracts: Take valerian tinctures or liquid extracts orally for a concentrated dose of its therapeutic effects. Add a few drops of valerian extract to water or juice and consume it as needed to ease anxiety or promote relaxation. Tinctures provide a convenient and potent way to experience valerian's calming benefits.

Capsules or Tablets: Take valerian supplements in capsule or tablet form for a standardized dose of its active compounds. Follow the manufacturer's dosage recommendations for optimal results.

Valerian supplements are particularly useful for individuals who prefer a convenient and consistent way to incorporate valerian into their routine.

Safety Considerations

Valerian is generally safe for most people when used appropriately. However, it may cause drowsiness or dizziness in some individuals, especially when taken in high doses or combined with other sedative medications. Pregnant or breastfeeding women, as well as individuals with liver disease or sensitivity to valerian, should consult with a healthcare professional before using valerian supplements.

Valerian, with its gentle yet effective calming properties, offers a natural solution for promoting relaxation, easing anxiety, and improving sleep quality. By harnessing the power of this remarkable herb, individuals can find solace in the midst of life's stresses, cultivate inner peace, and embrace restful sleep with open arms. With valerian as a trusted ally in the quest for tranquility, we journey toward a life of balance, harmony, and well-being, one peaceful night at a time.

Lemon Balm: Nature's Soothing Balm

Introduction

Lemon balm, with its refreshing citrus scent and gentle demeanor, emerges as a cherished herb in the realm of natural medicine. Revered for its calming properties and myriad health benefits, lemon balm offers a gentle yet effective remedy for promoting relaxation, easing stress, and uplifting the spirit. In this chapter, we delve into the remarkable properties of lemon balm and its role as nature's soothing balm.

Understanding Lemon Balm

Botanical Background: Lemon balm (Melissa officinalis) is a perennial herb belonging to the mint family (Lamiaceae) and is native to the Mediterranean region. It features aromatic, heart-shaped leaves with a distinct lemon scent and small white or pale pink flowers that attract bees and other pollinators. Lemon balm has been cultivated for centuries for its culinary, medicinal, and aromatic properties.

Medicinal Properties: Lemon balm is prized for its calming, antiviral, and mood-lifting properties, making it a versatile remedy for various health concerns. Its primary bioactive compounds include rosmarinic acid, citronellal, and flavonoids, which contribute to its therapeutic effects on the nervous system, immune system, and digestive system.

Harnessing the Power of Lemon Balm

Stress Relief: Lemon balm is renowned for its ability to reduce stress, anxiety, and nervous tension. It has mild sedative effects that help promote relaxation and induce a sense of calmness, making it an ideal remedy for individuals experiencing stress-related symptoms such as restlessness, irritability, or difficulty concentrating.

Mood Enhancement: Lemon balm has mood-lifting properties that can help improve mood and emotional well-being. It modulates neurotransmitter activity in the brain, including serotonin and gamma-aminobutyric acid (GABA), which play key roles in mood regulation and stress response. Lemon balm's uplifting effects can help soothe the mind and lift the spirits during times of emotional distress.

Digestive Support: Lemon balm has carminative and digestive properties that can help soothe digestive discomfort and promote healthy digestion. It may be beneficial for individuals experiencing symptoms such as bloating, gas, indigestion, or stomach cramps. Lemon balm's gentle calming effects extend to the digestive system, helping to ease tension and promote comfort.

How to Use Lemon Balm

Herbal Tea: Brew lemon balm leaves into a fragrant herbal tea by steeping them in hot water for 5-10 minutes. Strain the tea and drink it warm or chilled as a soothing and refreshing beverage. Lemon balm tea can be enjoyed on its own or combined with other herbs such as chamomile or lavender for added relaxation.

Tinctures and Extracts: Take lemon balm tinctures or liquid extracts orally for a concentrated dose of its therapeutic effects. Add a few drops of lemon balm extract to water or juice and consume it as needed to ease stress or promote relaxation. Tinctures provide a convenient and potent way to experience lemon balm's calming benefits.

Aromatherapy: Use lemon balm essential oil for aromatherapy by diffusing it in your home or workplace to create a calming and uplifting atmosphere. You can also add a few drops of lemon balm oil to a warm bath or massage oil for a relaxing and rejuvenating experience. Lemon balm's aromatic properties help soothe the mind and promote emotional well-being.

Safety Considerations

Lemon balm is generally safe for most people when used appropriately. However, it may cause mild side effects such as drowsiness or digestive upset in some individuals, especially when taken in high doses. Pregnant or breastfeeding women, as well as individuals with thyroid conditions or allergies to the mint family, should consult with a healthcare professional before using lemon balm supplements.

Lemon balm, with its gentle yet profound calming effects, offers a natural remedy for promoting relaxation, easing stress, and uplifting the spirit. By harnessing the power of this remarkable herb, individuals can find solace in the midst of life's challenges, cultivate inner peace, and embrace a sense of well-being from within. With lemon balm as a trusted ally in the quest for tranquility, we journey toward a life of balance, harmony, and vitality, one soothing sip at a time.

Passionflower: Nature's Tranquilizer

Introduction

Passionflower, with its intricate blooms and serene presence, emerges as a symbol of tranquility and relaxation in the world of herbal medicine. Revered for its calming properties and gentle sedative effects, passionflower offers a natural remedy for promoting restful sleep, easing anxiety, and soothing the mind. In this chapter, we explore the remarkable properties of passionflower and its role as nature's tranquilizer.

Understanding Passionflower

Botanical Background: Passionflower, scientifically known as Passiflora incarnata, is a climbing vine native to the southeastern United States and Central and South America. It features exotic flowers with striking colors and complex structures, resembling a miniature work of art.

Passionflower has a long history of use in traditional medicine for its sedative, anxiolytic, and hypnotic properties.

Medicinal Properties: Passionflower is prized for its calming effects on the nervous system and its ability to promote relaxation and improve sleep quality. Its primary bioactive compounds include flavonoids, alkaloids, and glycosides, which contribute to its therapeutic effects on neurotransmitter activity and stress response.

Harnessing the Power of Passionflower

Sleep Support: Passionflower is best known for its ability to promote restful sleep and alleviate insomnia. It helps reduce the time it takes to fall asleep, improve sleep quality, and enhance overall sleep duration, making it an effective alternative to conventional sleep aids. Passionflower works by increasing levels of gamma-aminobutyric acid (GABA), a neurotransmitter that promotes relaxation and regulates sleep-wake cycles.

Anxiety Relief: Passionflower has anxiolytic properties that help reduce feelings of anxiety, nervousness, and tension. It modulates neurotransmitter activity in the brain, including gamma-aminobutyric acid (GABA), serotonin, and dopamine, which play key roles in mood regulation and emotional well-being. Passionflower's calming effects can help soothe frazzled nerves and promote a sense of inner peace.

Muscle Relaxation: Passionflower has muscle-relaxant properties that can help ease tension and stiffness in the body. It may be beneficial for individuals experiencing muscle spasms, cramps, or discomfort associated with stress or physical exertion. Passionflower's calming effects extend beyond the mind to the muscles, promoting overall relaxation and comfort.

How to Use Passionflower

Herbal Tea: Brew dried passionflower leaves and flowers into a soothing herbal tea by steeping them in hot water for 5-10 minutes. Strain the tea and drink it before bedtime to promote relaxation and improve sleep quality. You can also combine passionflower with other calming herbs such as chamomile or lemon balm for added flavor and benefits.

Tinctures and Extracts: Take passionflower tinctures or liquid extracts orally for a concentrated dose of its therapeutic effects. Add a few drops of passionflower extract to water or juice and consume it as needed to ease anxiety or promote relaxation. Tinctures provide a convenient and potent way to experience passionflower's calming benefits.

Capsules or Tablets: Take passionflower supplements in capsule or tablet form for a standardized dose of its active compounds. Follow the manufacturer's dosage recommendations for optimal results. Passionflower supplements are particularly useful for individuals who prefer a convenient and consistent way to incorporate passionflower into their routine.

Safety Considerations

Passionflower is generally safe for most people when used appropriately. However, it may cause drowsiness or dizziness in some individuals, especially when taken in high doses or combined with other sedative medications. Pregnant or breastfeeding women, as well as individuals with liver disease or sensitivity to passionflower, should consult with a healthcare professional before using passionflower supplements.

Passionflower, with its gentle yet profound calming effects, offers a natural remedy for promoting relaxation, easing anxiety, and improving sleep quality. By harnessing the power of this remarkable herb, individuals can find solace in the midst of life's stresses, cultivate inner peace, and embrace restful sleep with open arms. With passionflower as a trusted ally in the quest for tranquility, we journey toward a life of balance, harmony, and well-being, one serene moment at a time.

Improving Sleep Quality: Herbal Remedies for Restful Nights

Introduction

In today's fast-paced world, achieving restful sleep has become increasingly challenging for many individuals. Poor sleep quality can have a profound impact on physical, mental, and emotional well-being, leading to fatigue, irritability, and impaired cognitive function. While various factors contribute to sleep disturbances, herbal medicine offers a natural and holistic approach to promoting relaxation, easing anxiety, and improving sleep quality. In this chapter, we explore the therapeutic potential of herbs in enhancing sleep quality and restoring restful nights.

Understanding Sleep Quality

The Importance of Sleep: Sleep is essential for overall health and well-being, playing a vital role in physical restoration, cognitive function, and emotional regulation. Quality sleep is characterized by sufficient duration, uninterrupted sleep cycles, and restorative rest, allowing the body and mind to recharge and rejuvenate for the day ahead.

Factors Affecting Sleep Quality: Sleep quality can be influenced by various factors, including stress, anxiety, poor sleep hygiene, lifestyle habits, and underlying health conditions. Stress and anxiety can disrupt sleep patterns and impair relaxation, while poor sleep hygiene, such as excessive screen time or irregular sleep schedules, can interfere with the body's natural circadian rhythm.

Herbal Support for Sleep Quality

Sedative Herbs: Certain herbs, such as valerian, passionflower, and lemon balm, have sedative properties that promote relaxation and induce sleep. They help calm the nervous system, reduce anxiety, and improve sleep onset and duration, making them valuable allies for individuals experiencing sleep disturbances or insomnia.

Adaptogens: Adaptogenic herbs, such as ashwagandha and rhodiola, help the body adapt to stress and promote resilience, which can indirectly improve sleep quality. By reducing stress levels and supporting adrenal gland function, adaptogens help regulate the body's stress response system and promote relaxation, leading to better sleep quality.

Nervines: Nervine herbs, including chamomile, lavender, and skullcap, have calming and soothing effects on the nervous system, making them ideal for promoting relaxation and easing anxiety before bedtime. They help quiet the mind, reduce tension, and prepare the body for restful sleep, improving overall sleep quality.

Incorporating Herbal Remedies into Bedtime Routine

Herbal Teas: Brew herbal teas using dried herbs or tea bags for a soothing and relaxing beverage before bedtime. Enjoy a cup of chamomile tea or valerian tea to promote relaxation and improve sleep quality. Experiment with different herbal blends to find the ones that work best for you.

Aromatherapy: Use essential oils derived from calming herbs such as lavender, bergamot, and chamomile for aromatherapy. Diffuse essential oils in your bedroom or add a few drops to a warm bath before bedtime to create a calming and relaxing atmosphere. Aromatherapy can help soothe the mind and promote restful sleep.

Tinctures and Extracts: Take herbal tinctures or liquid extracts orally for a concentrated dose of therapeutic herbs. Add a few drops of passionflower extract or lemon balm tincture to water or juice and consume it before bedtime to ease anxiety and promote relaxation. Tinctures provide a convenient and effective way to incorporate herbs into your bedtime routine.

Safety Considerations

While herbs are generally safe when used appropriately, it's essential to consult with a qualified healthcare practitioner before using herbal remedies, especially if you are pregnant, breastfeeding, or taking medications. Some herbs may interact with medications or have contraindications for certain individuals, so it's crucial to seek personalized guidance to ensure safe and effective use.

Improving sleep quality is essential for overall health and well-being, and herbal remedies offer a natural and holistic approach to achieving restful nights. By incorporating sedative herbs, adaptogens, and nervines into your bedtime routine, you can promote relaxation, ease anxiety, and improve sleep quality. With herbal remedies as allies in the quest for restful sleep, you can awaken feeling refreshed, rejuvenated, and ready to embrace the day ahead.

Chamomile: Nature's Calming Elixir

Introduction

In the realm of herbal medicine, few remedies are as cherished and beloved as chamomile. With its delicate flowers and soothing aroma, chamomile emerges as a gentle yet potent ally in promoting relaxation, easing tension, and supporting overall well-being. For centuries, this humble herb has been revered for its calming properties and myriad health benefits. In this chapter, we explore the remarkable properties of chamomile and its role as nature's calming elixir.

Understanding Chamomile

Botanical Background: Chamomile, scientifically known as Matricaria chamomilla or Chamaemelum nobile, is a flowering plant belonging to the Asteraceae family. It is native to Europe, Asia, and North Africa and is characterized by its daisy-like flowers with white petals and yellow centers. Chamomile has a long history of use in traditional medicine and is renowned for its soothing and healing properties.

Medicinal Properties: Chamomile is prized for its anti-inflammatory, antispasmodic, and sedative properties, making it a versatile remedy for various health concerns. Its primary bioactive compounds include chamazulene, apigenin, and bisabolol, which contribute to its therapeutic effects on the nervous system, digestive system, and skin.

Harnessing the Power of Chamomile

Stress Relief: Chamomile is best known for its ability to reduce stress, anxiety, and nervous tension. It has mild sedative effects that help promote relaxation and induce a sense of calmness, making it an ideal remedy for individuals experiencing stress-related symptoms such as restlessness, irritability, or difficulty concentrating.

Digestive Support: Chamomile has carminative and digestive properties that can help soothe digestive discomfort and promote healthy digestion. It may be beneficial for individuals experiencing symptoms such as bloating, gas, indigestion, or stomach cramps. Chamomile's gentle calming effects extend to the digestive system, helping to ease tension and promote comfort.

Skin Soothing: Chamomile has anti-inflammatory and antiseptic properties that make it a valuable remedy for skin conditions such as eczema, psoriasis, and minor wounds. It helps reduce inflammation, soothe irritation, and promote healing, making it a popular ingredient in skincare products such as creams, lotions, and ointments.

How to Use Chamomile

Herbal Tea: Brew dried chamomile flowers into a soothing herbal tea by steeping them in hot water for 5-10 minutes. Strain the tea and drink it warm or chilled as a calming and refreshing beverage. Chamomile tea can be enjoyed on its own or combined with other herbs such as lavender or lemon balm for added flavor and benefits.

Tinctures and Extracts: Take chamomile tinctures or liquid extracts orally for a concentrated dose of its therapeutic effects. Add a few drops of chamomile extract to water or juice and consume it as needed to ease anxiety or promote relaxation. Tinctures provide a convenient and potent way to experience chamomile's calming benefits.

Topical Applications: Apply chamomile-infused creams, lotions, or ointments topically to soothe skin irritation, inflammation, or minor wounds. Chamomile can help reduce redness, itching, and swelling, making it a gentle and effective remedy for various skin conditions. Apply the topical preparation as needed to the affected area and gently massage it into the skin.

Safety Considerations

Chamomile is generally safe for most people when used appropriately. However, individuals with allergies to plants in the Asteraceae family, such as ragweed, marigolds, or daisies, may experience allergic reactions to chamomile. Pregnant or breastfeeding women, as well as individuals taking blood-thinning medications or sedatives, should consult with a healthcare professional before using chamomile supplements.

Chamomile, with its gentle yet profound calming effects, offers a natural remedy for promoting relaxation, easing tension, and supporting overall well-being. By harnessing the power of this remarkable herb, individuals can find solace in the midst of life's stresses, cultivate inner peace, and embrace a sense of well-being from within. With chamomile as a trusted ally in the quest for tranquility, we journey toward a life of balance, harmony, and vitality, one soothing sip at a time.

Lavender: Nature's Aromatic Healer

Introduction

Lavender, with its enchanting fragrance and vibrant blooms, emerges as a symbol of tranquility and healing in the world of herbal medicine. Revered for its calming properties and myriad health benefits, lavender offers a natural remedy for promoting relaxation, easing stress, and supporting overall well-being. In this chapter, we explore the remarkable properties of lavender and its role as nature's aromatic healer.

Understanding Lavender

Botanical Background: Lavender, scientifically known as Lavandula angustifolia, is a flowering plant native to the Mediterranean region and is cultivated worldwide for its aromatic flowers and essential oil. It is characterized by slender stems, narrow leaves, and clusters of fragrant purple or blue flowers. Lavender has been used for centuries in traditional medicine, aromatherapy, and culinary applications.

Medicinal Properties: Lavender is prized for its calming, antiseptic, and analgesic properties, making it a versatile remedy for various health concerns. Its primary bioactive compounds include linalool, linalyl acetate, and camphor, which contribute to its therapeutic effects on the nervous system, skin, and respiratory system.

Harnessing the Power of Lavender

Stress Relief: Lavender is best known for its ability to reduce stress, anxiety, and nervous tension. It has a calming effect on the nervous system, helping to promote relaxation and induce a sense of tranquility. Lavender's aromatic compounds interact with neurotransmitters in the brain, including serotonin and gamma-aminobutyric acid (GABA), which play key roles in mood regulation and stress response.

Sleep Support: Lavender is renowned for its sleep-promoting properties and its ability to improve sleep quality. Inhalation of lavender essential oil or the use of lavender sachets in the bedroom can help create a calming and relaxing atmosphere conducive to restful sleep. Lavender's soothing aroma helps quiet the mind, reduce bedtime anxiety, and promote deep, rejuvenating sleep.

Skin Healing: Lavender has antiseptic and anti-inflammatory properties that make it a valuable remedy for various skin conditions. It can help soothe irritation, reduce redness and swelling, and promote healing of minor wounds, burns, and insect bites. Lavender essential oil can be diluted in a carrier oil and applied topically to the affected area for gentle and effective skin care.

How to Use Lavender

Aromatherapy: Use lavender essential oil for aromatherapy by diffusing it in your home or workplace to create a calming and uplifting atmosphere. Lavender's soothing aroma helps reduce stress, anxiety, and tension, promoting a sense of well-being and relaxation. Diffuse lavender essential oil for 15-30 minutes before bedtime to prepare the mind and body for sleep.

Topical Applications: Apply diluted lavender essential oil topically to the skin for various health and beauty benefits. Lavender oil can be added to carrier oils such as coconut oil or jojoba oil and used for massage, moisturizing, or spot treatment of skin conditions. Lavender-infused creams, lotions, and balms are also available for convenient application.

Herbal Baths: Add a few drops of lavender essential oil to a warm bath for a luxurious and relaxing soak. Lavender-scented baths help soothe sore muscles, relieve tension, and promote relaxation of the body and mind. Combine lavender essential oil with Epsom salts or bath bubbles for added therapeutic benefits.

Safety Considerations

Lavender is generally safe for most people when used appropriately. However, some individuals may experience allergic reactions or skin sensitivities to lavender essential oil. Pregnant or breastfeeding women, as well as individuals with allergies or sensitivities to fragrances, should consult with a healthcare professional before using lavender essential oil.

Lavender, with its enchanting fragrance and therapeutic properties, offers a natural remedy for promoting relaxation, easing stress, and supporting overall well-being. By harnessing the power of this remarkable herb, individuals can find solace in the midst of life's challenges, cultivate inner peace, and embrace a sense of well-being from within. With lavender as a trusted ally in the quest for tranquility, we journey toward a life of balance, harmony, and vitality, one fragrant breath at a time.

Hops: Nature's Sedative

Introduction

In the world of herbal medicine, hops emerge as a powerful yet underappreciated remedy for promoting relaxation and inducing sleep. With their distinctive aroma and bitter flavor, hops have been used for centuries to create beer, but their therapeutic properties extend far beyond the brewing process. In this chapter, we delve into the remarkable properties of hops and their role as nature's sedative.

Understanding Hops

Botanical Background: Hops, scientifically known as Humulus lupulus, are the female flowers of the hop plant, a perennial vine belonging to the Cannabaceae family. Native to Europe, Asia, and North America, hops are cultivated worldwide for their use in brewing beer and their medicinal properties. Hops are characterized by their green, cone-shaped flowers and resinous glands, which contain the plant's bioactive compounds.

Medicinal Properties: Hops are prized for their sedative, anxiolytic, and hypnotic properties, making them a valuable remedy for promoting relaxation and improving sleep quality. The primary bioactive compounds in hops include bitter acids, essential oils, and flavonoids, which contribute to their therapeutic effects on the nervous system and mood regulation.

Harnessing the Power of Hops

Sleep Support: Hops are best known for their sleep-promoting properties and their ability to improve sleep quality. They contain natural sedative compounds that help calm the nervous system, reduce anxiety, and induce feelings of relaxation. Hops can be used alone or in combination with other sleep-promoting herbs, such as valerian or chamomile, to create a potent remedy for insomnia and sleep disturbances.

Anxiety Relief: Hops have anxiolytic effects that help reduce feelings of stress, nervousness, and tension. The bioactive compounds in hops interact with neurotransmitters in the brain, including gamma-aminobutyric acid (GABA), which plays a key role in mood regulation and stress response. Hops can help quiet the mind, soothe frazzled nerves, and promote a sense of calmness and well-being.

Digestive Support: Hops have digestive properties that can help soothe gastrointestinal discomfort and promote healthy digestion. They contain bitter acids that stimulate digestive juices and enzymes, aiding in the digestion of food and alleviating symptoms such as bloating, gas, and indigestion. Hops can be used as a digestive tonic before or after meals to support optimal digestive function.

How to Use Hops

Herbal Tea: Brew dried hops flowers into a soothing herbal tea by steeping them in hot water for 5-10 minutes. Strain the tea and drink it warm before bedtime to promote relaxation and improve sleep quality. You can also combine hops with other calming herbs such as chamomile or lavender for added flavor and benefits.

Tinctures and Extracts: Take hops tinctures or liquid extracts orally for a concentrated dose of its therapeutic effects. Add a few drops of hops extract to water or juice and consume it as needed to ease anxiety or promote relaxation. Tinctures provide a convenient and potent way to experience hops' sedative benefits.

Pillow Sachets: Fill a small cloth sachet with dried hops flowers and place it inside your pillowcase to enjoy the soothing aroma of hops as you sleep. The gentle scent of hops can help calm the mind, reduce bedtime anxiety, and promote restful sleep.

Safety Considerations

Hops are generally safe for most people when used appropriately. However, they may cause drowsiness or dizziness in some individuals, especially when taken in high doses or combined with other sedative medications. Pregnant or breastfeeding women, as well as individuals with hormone-sensitive conditions or depression, should consult with a healthcare professional before using hops supplements.

Hops, with their sedative properties and soothing aroma, offer a natural remedy for promoting relaxation, easing anxiety, and improving sleep quality. By harnessing the power of this remarkable herb, individuals can find solace in the midst of life's stresses, cultivate inner peace, and embrace restful sleep with open arms. With hops as a trusted ally in the quest for tranquility, we journey toward a life of balance, harmony, and vitality, one tranquil night at a time.

Skullcap: Nature's Stress Reliever

Introduction

In the world of herbal medicine, skullcap stands out as a potent yet gentle remedy for promoting relaxation and easing stress. With its delicate flowers and calming properties, skullcap offers a natural solution for soothing frazzled nerves and restoring inner peace. In this chapter, we explore the remarkable properties of skullcap and its role as nature's stress reliever.

Understanding Skullcap

Botanical Background: Skullcap, scientifically known as Scutellaria lateriflora, is a perennial herb native to North America, where it grows in wetlands, meadows, and along stream banks. It belongs to the mint family (Lamiaceae) and is characterized by its slender stems, small blue or purple flowers, and scallop-shaped leaves. Skullcap has a long history of use in traditional medicine for its calming and nervine properties.

Medicinal Properties: Skullcap is prized for its anxiolytic, sedative, and nervine properties, making it a valuable remedy for promoting relaxation and easing nervous tension. The primary bioactive compounds in skullcap include flavonoids, phenolic acids, and volatile oils, which contribute to its therapeutic effects on the nervous system and mood regulation.

Harnessing the Power of Skullcap

Stress Relief: Skullcap is best known for its ability to reduce stress, anxiety, and nervous tension. It has a calming effect on the nervous system, helping to soothe frazzled nerves and promote a sense of tranquility. Skullcap's bioactive compounds interact with neurotransmitters in the brain, including gamma-aminobutyric acid (GABA), which plays a key role in mood regulation and stress response.

Sleep Support: Skullcap has sleep-promoting properties that can help improve sleep quality and duration. By calming the mind and relaxing the body, skullcap helps prepare the mind for restful sleep. Skullcap can be used alone or in combination with other sedative herbs, such as valerian or passionflower, to create a potent remedy for insomnia and sleep disturbances.

Nervine Support: Skullcap acts as a nervine tonic, supporting the overall health and function of the nervous system. It helps strengthen the nervous system, improve resilience to stress, and enhance mental clarity and focus. Skullcap's nervine properties make it a valuable ally for individuals experiencing nervous exhaustion, burnout, or cognitive fatigue.

How to Use Skullcap

Herbal Tea: Brew dried skullcap leaves and flowers into a soothing herbal tea by steeping them in hot water for 5-10 minutes. Strain the tea and drink it warm before bedtime or during times of stress to promote relaxation and ease anxiety. Skullcap tea can be enjoyed on its own or combined with other calming herbs such as chamomile or lemon balm for added flavor and benefits.

Tinctures and Extracts: Take skullcap tinctures or liquid extracts orally for a concentrated dose of its therapeutic effects. Add a few drops of skullcap extract to water or juice and consume it as needed to ease anxiety or promote relaxation. Tinctures provide a convenient and potent way to experience skullcap's calming benefits.

Capsules or Tablets: Take skullcap supplements in capsule or tablet form for a standardized dose of its active compounds. Follow the manufacturer's dosage recommendations for optimal results. Skullcap supplements are particularly useful for individuals who prefer a convenient and consistent way to incorporate skullcap into their routine.

Safety Considerations

Skullcap is generally safe for most people when used appropriately. However, it may cause drowsiness or dizziness in some individuals, especially when taken in high doses or combined with other sedative medications. Pregnant or breastfeeding women, as well as individuals with liver disease or sensitivity to skullcap, should consult with a healthcare professional before using skullcap supplements.

Skullcap, with its calming properties and gentle nature, offers a natural remedy for promoting relaxation, easing stress, and supporting overall well-being. By harnessing the power of this remarkable herb, individuals can find solace in the midst of life's challenges, cultivate inner peace, and embrace a sense of tranquility from within. With skullcap as a trusted ally in the quest for stress relief, we journey toward a life of balance, harmony, and vitality, one serene moment at a time.

Enhancing Cognitive Function: Herbal Allies for Mental Clarity

Introduction

In the pursuit of optimal well-being, cognitive function plays a vital role in our daily lives. From sharp focus to mental agility, our ability to think clearly and retain information profoundly impacts our productivity and quality of life. While various factors can influence cognitive performance, herbal medicine offers a natural and holistic approach to enhancing mental clarity and cognitive function. In this chapter, we explore the remarkable properties of herbs and their role in supporting brain health and cognitive vitality.

Understanding Cognitive Function

The Importance of Cognitive Health: Cognitive function encompasses a range of mental processes, including memory, attention, reasoning, and problem-solving. Optimal cognitive function is essential for performing everyday tasks, navigating complex situations, and maintaining overall mental well-being. Factors such as stress, aging, poor nutrition, and lifestyle habits can affect cognitive performance and contribute to cognitive decline over time.

Herbal Support for Cognitive Function: Herbal remedies have been used for centuries to support brain health and enhance cognitive function. Certain herbs contain bioactive compounds that nourish the brain, improve blood flow, reduce inflammation, and protect against oxidative stress, all of which contribute to enhanced cognitive performance and mental clarity.

Herbal Allies for Cognitive Enhancement

Ginkgo Biloba: Ginkgo biloba is a renowned herb for cognitive enhancement, known for its ability to improve memory, concentration, and overall cognitive function. It enhances blood flow to the brain, increases oxygenation, and protects neurons from oxidative damage, promoting mental clarity and alertness. Ginkgo biloba is particularly beneficial for individuals experiencing age-related cognitive decline or memory impairment.

Bacopa Monnieri: Bacopa monnieri, also known as Brahmi, is an Ayurvedic herb prized for its cognitive-enhancing properties. It supports memory retention, learning ability, and mental focus by modulating neurotransmitter activity and promoting synaptic plasticity. Bacopa monnieri is a valuable ally for students, professionals, and individuals seeking to improve cognitive performance and academic achievement.

Rosemary: Rosemary is a culinary herb with cognitive-enhancing properties, known for its ability to improve memory, concentration, and mental clarity. It contains compounds such as rosmarinic acid and carnosic acid, which have neuroprotective effects and enhance cognitive function. Rosemary essential oil can be used in aromatherapy to stimulate cognitive function and enhance alertness.

Incorporating Herbs into Daily Routine

Herbal Teas: Brew herbal teas using dried herbs or tea bags for a convenient and enjoyable way to incorporate herbs into your daily routine. Enjoy a cup of ginkgo biloba tea or bacopa monnieri tea before studying or working to enhance cognitive function and mental clarity. Experiment with different herbal blends to find the ones that work best for you.

Tinctures and Extracts: Take herbal tinctures or liquid extracts orally for a concentrated dose of therapeutic herbs. Add a few drops of ginkgo biloba extract or rosemary tincture to water or juice and consume it as needed to support cognitive function and mental alertness. Tinctures provide a convenient and potent way to experience the benefits of herbs.

Supplements: Take herbal supplements in capsule or tablet form for a standardized dose of active compounds. Follow the manufacturer's dosage recommendations for optimal results. Herbal supplements are particularly useful for individuals who prefer a convenient and consistent way to incorporate herbs into their daily routine.

Safety Considerations

While herbs are generally safe when used appropriately, it's essential to consult with a qualified healthcare practitioner before using herbal remedies, especially if you are pregnant, breastfeeding, or taking medications. Some herbs may interact with medications or have contraindications for certain individuals, so it's crucial to seek personalized guidance to ensure safe and effective use.

Enhancing cognitive function is essential for maintaining mental clarity, focus, and productivity in our daily lives. By harnessing the power of herbs, individuals can support brain health, enhance cognitive performance, and promote overall mental well-being. With herbal allies as companions in the quest for cognitive enhancement, we journey toward a life of clarity, creativity, and cognitive vitality, one mindful moment at a time.

Ginkgo Biloba: Nature's Memory Enhancer

Introduction

In the quest for optimal cognitive function and mental clarity, few herbs have garnered as much attention and acclaim as ginkgo biloba. Revered for its ability to support memory, concentration, and overall brain health, ginkgo biloba has stood the test of time as a potent ally for cognitive enhancement. In this chapter, we delve into the remarkable properties of ginkgo biloba and its role as nature's memory enhancer.

Understanding Ginkgo Biloba

Botanical Background: Ginkgo biloba, also known as the maidenhair tree, is one of the oldest living tree species on Earth, with a lineage dating back millions of years. Native to China, ginkgo biloba is now cultivated worldwide for its medicinal properties and ornamental value. The tree produces distinctive fan-shaped leaves and small, fleshy seeds that contain bioactive compounds used in herbal medicine.

Medicinal Properties: Ginkgo biloba is prized for its cognitive-enhancing properties, particularly its ability to improve memory, concentration, and overall brain function. The primary bioactive compounds in ginkgo biloba include flavonoids, terpenoids, and ginkgolides, which contribute to its neuroprotective, antioxidant, and vasodilatory effects on the brain.

Harnessing the Power of Ginkgo Biloba

Memory Enhancement: Ginkgo biloba is best known for its ability to support memory and cognitive function, making it a popular supplement for students, professionals, and older adults seeking to maintain mental sharpness. It enhances blood flow to the brain, improves oxygenation, and protects neurons from oxidative damage, which promotes memory retention and cognitive performance.

Focus and Concentration: Ginkgo biloba can help improve focus, concentration, and mental clarity by enhancing neurotransmitter activity and optimizing brain function. It helps reduce mental fatigue, enhance alertness, and improve cognitive processing speed, making it a valuable ally for tasks requiring sustained attention and mental acuity.

Brain Health Support: Ginkgo biloba has neuroprotective properties that help support overall brain health and resilience to age-related cognitive decline. It protects neurons from oxidative stress, reduces inflammation, and enhances synaptic plasticity, which supports cognitive longevity and healthy aging of the brain.

How to Use Ginkgo Biloba

Standardized Extracts: Take ginkgo biloba supplements in standardized extract form for a consistent dose of active compounds. Follow the manufacturer's dosage recommendations for optimal results. Ginkgo biloba supplements are available in capsules, tablets, and liquid extracts, providing a convenient and reliable way to incorporate ginkgo biloba into your daily routine.

Herbal Tea: Brew ginkgo biloba tea using dried ginkgo leaves for a soothing and refreshing beverage. Steep the leaves in hot water for 5-10 minutes, then strain and enjoy the tea warm or chilled. Ginkgo biloba tea can be consumed daily to support cognitive function and overall brain health.

Topical Applications: Apply ginkgo biloba extract topically to the scalp as a natural remedy for promoting hair growth and scalp health. Ginkgo biloba extract helps improve circulation to the scalp, stimulate hair follicles, and nourish the hair and scalp with essential nutrients, promoting thicker, healthier hair growth.

Safety Considerations

Ginkgo biloba is generally safe for most people when used appropriately. However, it may interact with certain medications, including blood thinners, antidepressants, and anticonvulsants, so it's essential to consult with a healthcare professional before using ginkgo biloba supplements, especially if you are taking medications or have underlying health conditions.

Ginkgo biloba, with its memory-enhancing properties and neuroprotective effects, offers a natural solution for supporting cognitive function and brain health. By harnessing the power of this remarkable herb, individuals can maintain mental sharpness, enhance memory retention, and promote overall cognitive vitality. With ginkgo biloba as a trusted ally in the quest for optimal brain function, we journey toward a life of clarity, creativity, and cognitive well-being, one mindful moment at a time.

Rosemary: Nature's Cognitive Stimulant

Introduction

In the world of herbal medicine, few plants evoke the senses and invigorate the mind like rosemary. With its aromatic fragrance and culinary versatility, rosemary has long been revered for its therapeutic properties and cognitive-enhancing effects. In this chapter, we explore the remarkable attributes of rosemary and its role as nature's cognitive stimulant.

Understanding Rosemary

Botanical Background: Rosemary, scientifically known as Rosmarinus officinalis, is an evergreen shrub native to the Mediterranean region but cultivated worldwide for its culinary and medicinal uses. It belongs to the mint family (Lamiaceae) and is characterized by its needle-like leaves, small blue flowers, and woody stems. Rosemary has a long history of use in traditional medicine and culinary traditions.

Medicinal Properties: Rosemary is prized for its cognitive-enhancing properties, particularly its ability to improve memory, concentration, and overall brain function. The primary bioactive compounds in rosemary include rosmarinic acid, carnosic acid, and essential oils, which contribute to its neuroprotective, antioxidant, and stimulant effects on the brain.

Harnessing the Power of Rosemary

Memory Enhancement: Rosemary is best known for its memory-enhancing effects, making it a popular herb for students, professionals, and older adults seeking to maintain cognitive function. Inhalation of rosemary essential oil or the use of rosemary-infused products can help improve memory retention, recall, and overall cognitive performance.

Mental Clarity: Rosemary has stimulating properties that help enhance mental clarity, focus, and alertness. Its invigorating aroma can help sharpen the mind, improve concentration, and boost productivity, making it an ideal herb for studying, working, or engaging in mentally demanding tasks.

Neuroprotective Effects: Rosemary has neuroprotective properties that help support overall brain health and resilience to age-related cognitive decline. It protects neurons from oxidative stress, reduces inflammation, and enhances synaptic plasticity, which supports cognitive longevity and healthy aging of the brain.

How to Use Rosemary

Aromatherapy: Use rosemary essential oil in aromatherapy to stimulate cognitive function and enhance mental clarity. Diffuse rosemary essential oil in your home or workplace to create a stimulating and uplifting atmosphere. Alternatively, add a few drops of rosemary essential oil to a warm bath or massage oil for a rejuvenating and invigorating experience.

Herbal Teas: Brew rosemary tea using dried rosemary leaves for a refreshing and aromatic beverage. Steep the leaves in hot water for 5-10 minutes, then strain and enjoy the tea warm or chilled. Rosemary tea can be consumed daily to support cognitive function and overall brain health.

Topical Applications: Apply rosemary-infused products topically to the skin for various health and beauty benefits. Rosemary essential oil can be diluted in a carrier oil and used for massage, skincare, or scalp treatments. Rosemary-infused creams, lotions, and hair care products are also available for convenient application.

Safety Considerations

Rosemary is generally safe for most people when used appropriately. However, individuals with allergies to plants in the Lamiaceae family, such as mint, basil, or oregano, may experience allergic reactions to rosemary. Pregnant or breastfeeding women, as well as individuals with epilepsy or high blood pressure, should consult with a healthcare professional before using rosemary supplements or essential oil.

Rosemary, with its cognitive-enhancing properties and stimulating effects, offers a natural solution for promoting mental clarity, focus, and overall brain health. By harnessing the power of this remarkable herb, individuals can sharpen their minds, enhance cognitive performance, and support optimal brain function. With rosemary as a trusted ally in the quest for cognitive vitality, we journey toward a life of clarity, creativity, and cognitive well-being, one aromatic breath at a time.

Bacopa: Nature's Brain Booster

Introduction

In the realm of herbal medicine, Bacopa monnieri, commonly known as Bacopa or Brahmi, stands out as a revered herb with profound effects on cognitive function and mental well-being. With its rich history in Ayurvedic tradition and modern scientific validation, Bacopa has earned a reputation as a potent brain tonic and memory enhancer. In this chapter, we explore the remarkable properties of Bacopa and its role as nature's brain booster.

Understanding Bacopa

Botanical Background: Bacopa monnieri is a perennial herb native to the wetlands of Asia, particularly India, where it has been used for centuries in traditional Ayurvedic medicine. It belongs to the plantain family (Plantaginaceae) and is characterized by its succulent leaves, small white flowers, and creeping habit. Bacopa is prized for its cognitive-enhancing properties and adaptogenic effects on the nervous system.

Medicinal Properties: Bacopa is renowned for its cognitive-enhancing and neuroprotective properties, making it a valuable remedy for improving memory, concentration, and overall brain function. The primary bioactive compounds in Bacopa include bacosides, saponins, and flavonoids, which have been shown to support synaptic plasticity, enhance neurotransmitter activity, and protect neurons from oxidative stress.

Harnessing the Power of Bacopa

Memory Enhancement: Bacopa is best known for its memory-enhancing effects, particularly its ability to improve memory retention, learning ability, and cognitive function. It enhances synaptic communication between neurons, promotes the growth of dendrites and axons, and increases the production of key neurotransmitters involved in memory formation, such as acetylcholine.

Focus and Concentration: Bacopa helps improve focus, concentration, and mental clarity by modulating neurotransmitter activity and optimizing brain function. It reduces stress-induced cognitive impairments, enhances attentional control, and promotes sustained mental performance, making it an ideal herb for students, professionals, and individuals seeking to improve cognitive performance.

Neuroprotective Effects: Bacopa has neuroprotective properties that help support overall brain health and resilience to age-related cognitive decline. It protects neurons from oxidative stress, reduces inflammation, and enhances neuronal plasticity, which supports cognitive longevity and healthy aging of the brain.

How to Use Bacopa

Herbal Supplements: Take Bacopa supplements in capsule or tablet form for a standardized dose of active compounds. Follow the manufacturer's dosage recommendations for optimal results. Bacopa supplements are available in various strengths and formulations, providing a convenient and reliable way to incorporate Bacopa into your daily routine.

Herbal Teas: Brew Bacopa tea using dried Bacopa leaves for a soothing and refreshing beverage. Steep the leaves in hot water for 5-10 minutes, then strain and enjoy the tea warm or chilled. Bacopa tea can be consumed daily to support cognitive function and overall brain health.

Tinctures and Extracts: Take Bacopa tinctures or liquid extracts orally for a concentrated dose of therapeutic compounds. Add a few drops of Bacopa extract to water or juice and consume it as needed to support cognitive function and mental well-being. Tinctures provide a convenient and potent way to experience the benefits of Bacopa.

Safety Considerations

Bacopa is generally safe for most people when used appropriately. However, it may cause mild gastrointestinal discomfort in some individuals, especially when taken in high doses. Pregnant or breastfeeding women, as well as individuals with thyroid disorders or epilepsy, should consult with a healthcare professional before using Bacopa supplements.

Bacopa, with its cognitive-enhancing properties and neuroprotective effects, offers a natural solution for supporting brain health, memory retention, and overall cognitive function. By harnessing the power of this remarkable herb, individuals can sharpen their minds, enhance mental clarity, and promote cognitive vitality. With Bacopa as a trusted ally in the quest for optimal brain function, we journey toward a life of clarity, creativity, and cognitive well-being, one mindful moment at a time.

Rhodiola: Nature's Stress Reliever

Introduction

In the fast-paced modern world, stress has become an inevitable part of daily life, taking a toll on our mental and physical well-being. In the quest for balance and resilience, Rhodiola rosea emerges as a potent herbal ally, revered for its ability to combat stress, enhance mood, and promote overall vitality. In this chapter, we delve into the remarkable properties of Rhodiola and its role as nature's stress reliever.

Understanding Rhodiola

Botanical Background: Rhodiola rosea, commonly known as Rhodiola or Arctic root, is a perennial herb native to the mountainous regions of Europe, Asia, and North America. It belongs to the Crassulaceae family and is characterized by its succulent leaves, yellow flowers, and adaptogenic properties. Rhodiola has a long history of use in traditional medicine, particularly in Siberian and Scandinavian cultures, where it was prized for its ability to increase stamina and resilience to stress.

Medicinal Properties: Rhodiola is revered for its adaptogenic, antidepressant, and neuroprotective properties, making it a valuable remedy for combating stress, enhancing mood, and supporting overall well-being. The primary bioactive compounds in Rhodiola include rosavins, salidroside, and polyphenols, which have been shown to modulate stress hormone levels, improve neurotransmitter activity, and protect against oxidative stress.

Harnessing the Power of Rhodiola

Stress Relief: Rhodiola is best known for its stress-relieving effects, particularly its ability to reduce the body's response to stressors and promote a sense of calmness and well-being. It helps regulate cortisol levels, the body's primary stress hormone, and modulates the stress response system, helping individuals adapt to stressful situations more effectively.

Mood Enhancement: Rhodiola has mood-enhancing properties that help alleviate symptoms of depression, anxiety, and low mood. It increases the availability of neurotransmitters such as serotonin, dopamine, and norepinephrine, which play key roles in mood regulation and emotional well-being. Rhodiola can help uplift the spirits, improve resilience to stress, and enhance overall mood.

Energy and Vitality: Rhodiola helps increase energy levels, enhance stamina, and improve physical performance by optimizing mitochondrial function and oxygen utilization in the body. It helps combat fatigue, increase endurance, and promote overall vitality, making it a valuable herb for athletes, students, and individuals with demanding lifestyles.

How to Use Rhodiola

Herbal Supplements: Take Rhodiola supplements in capsule or tablet form for a standardized dose of active compounds. Follow the manufacturer's dosage recommendations for optimal results. Rhodiola supplements are available in various strengths and formulations, providing a convenient and reliable way to incorporate Rhodiola into your daily routine.

Herbal Tea: Brew Rhodiola tea using dried Rhodiola root for a soothing and invigorating beverage. Steep the root in hot water for 5-10 minutes, then strain and enjoy the tea warm or chilled. Rhodiola tea can be consumed daily to support stress relief, mood enhancement, and overall vitality.

Tinctures and Extracts: Take Rhodiola tinctures or liquid extracts orally for a concentrated dose of therapeutic compounds. Add a few drops of Rhodiola extract to water or juice and consume it as needed to support stress relief and mood enhancement. Tinctures provide a convenient and potent way to experience the benefits of Rhodiola.

Safety Considerations

Rhodiola is generally safe for most people when used appropriately. However, it may cause mild side effects such as dry mouth, dizziness, or gastrointestinal discomfort in some individuals, especially when taken in high doses. Pregnant or breastfeeding women, as well as individuals with bipolar disorder or autoimmune conditions, should consult with a healthcare professional before using Rhodiola supplements.

Rhodiola, with its stress-relieving properties and mood-enhancing effects, offers a natural solution for promoting resilience, vitality, and emotional well-being. By harnessing the power of this remarkable herb, individuals can combat stress, enhance mood, and cultivate a sense of balance and vitality in their lives. With Rhodiola as a trusted ally in the quest for stress relief, we journey toward a life of resilience, vitality, and emotional well-being, one mindful breath at a time.

Introduction to Women's Health: Nurturing Wellness Across Lifetimes

Women's health encompasses a vast spectrum of physical, mental, and emotional well-being, intricately woven into the fabric of life's journey. From adolescence to menopause and beyond, the unique health needs of women evolve and shape their experiences, resilience, and vitality. In this exploration of women's health, we embark on a journey to understand the complexities, challenges, and triumphs that define the female experience.

Understanding Women's Health

A Holistic Perspective: Women's health extends far beyond reproductive concerns, encompassing a myriad of interconnected factors, including hormonal balance, emotional well-being, nutritional needs, and preventative care. A holistic approach to women's health recognizes the interplay of these elements and seeks to nurture wellness in all aspects of life.

Lifecycle Transitions: From the onset of puberty to the transition through menopause and beyond, women undergo a series of transformative milestones that profoundly impact their health and vitality. Each stage brings unique challenges and opportunities for growth, requiring personalized care and support to navigate with grace and resilience.

Exploring Key Health Topics

Reproductive Health: Reproductive health is a cornerstone of women's well-being, encompassing menstrual health, contraception, fertility, pregnancy, and childbirth. Understanding the intricacies of reproductive physiology and accessing comprehensive reproductive healthcare are essential components of women's health empowerment.

Hormonal Balance: Hormonal fluctuations play a significant role in women's health, influencing everything from mood and energy levels to reproductive function and bone health. Balancing hormones through lifestyle modifications, nutritional support, and targeted interventions can optimize women's health and vitality throughout life.

Mental and Emotional Wellness: Mental and emotional health are integral aspects of women's well-being, influencing overall quality of life, resilience, and fulfillment. Addressing stress, anxiety, depression, and other mental health concerns with compassion and support is essential for nurturing emotional wellness and promoting thriving.

Preventative Care: Prevention is the cornerstone of women's health, empowering individuals to take proactive steps to maintain wellness and prevent disease. Regular screenings, vaccinations, healthy lifestyle choices, and self-care practices are essential components of preventative care for women of all ages.

Empowering Women's Health

Education and Advocacy: Empowering women's health begins with education and advocacy, equipping individuals with the knowledge, resources, and support they need to make informed decisions about their health and well-being. By raising awareness, challenging stigma, and advocating for equitable access to healthcare, we can create a world where all women have the opportunity to thrive.

Community and Support: Building supportive communities and fostering meaningful connections are vital aspects of women's health empowerment. By creating spaces for sharing experiences, offering support, and celebrating resilience, we can cultivate a culture of solidarity, compassion, and healing.

Women's health is a dynamic and multifaceted journey, guided by the principles of empowerment, resilience, and holistic well-being. By embracing a comprehensive approach that honors the diverse needs and experiences of women, we can nurture wellness across lifetimes, fostering a world where every woman has the opportunity to thrive in body, mind, and spirit.

Menstrual Health and PMS: Nurturing Wellness Through the Menstrual Cycle

Introduction

Menstruation is a natural and essential aspect of reproductive health, marking the cyclical rhythm of a woman's body. Yet, for many women, menstrual health encompasses far more than the physical process itself. It involves a delicate balance of hormones, emotions, and physical well-being, with each menstrual cycle offering insight into overall health and vitality. In this chapter, we explore the intricacies of menstrual health and premenstrual syndrome (PMS), shedding light on the challenges and opportunities for nurturing wellness throughout the menstrual cycle.

Understanding Menstrual Health

The Menstrual Cycle: The menstrual cycle is a complex interplay of hormonal fluctuations that prepare the body for potential pregnancy. It typically lasts around 28 days, although variations are common. The menstrual cycle consists of four phases: menstruation, the follicular phase, ovulation, and the luteal phase, each governed by shifting levels of estrogen, progesterone, and other hormones.

Menstrual Health Indicators: Menstrual health serves as a barometer of overall well-being, reflecting the body's hormonal balance, reproductive function, and general health. Regular menstrual cycles, minimal discomfort, and balanced mood are signs of optimal menstrual health, while irregular cycles, severe pain, and emotional disturbances may indicate underlying imbalances or health concerns.

Exploring Premenstrual Syndrome (PMS)

Understanding PMS: Premenstrual syndrome (PMS) refers to a combination of physical, emotional, and behavioral symptoms that occur in the days leading up to menstruation. Common symptoms include mood swings, irritability, fatigue, bloating, breast tenderness, and headaches. While mild PMS symptoms are normal for many women, severe symptoms can significantly impact quality of life and require intervention.

Hormonal Imbalances: PMS is thought to arise from hormonal imbalances, particularly fluctuations in estrogen and progesterone levels during the luteal phase of the menstrual cycle. These hormonal shifts can affect neurotransmitter activity in the brain, leading to mood disturbances, fluid retention, and other PMS symptoms.

Managing Menstrual Health and PMS

Lifestyle Modifications: Lifestyle modifications play a key role in managing menstrual health and reducing PMS symptoms. Regular exercise, balanced nutrition, stress management techniques, and adequate sleep can help regulate hormones, reduce inflammation, and support overall well-being throughout the menstrual cycle.

Nutritional Support: Certain nutrients and dietary supplements may help alleviate PMS symptoms and promote menstrual health. Calcium, magnesium, vitamin B6, and omega-3 fatty acids have been shown to have beneficial effects on mood, cramping, and bloating associated with PMS.

Herbal Remedies: Herbal remedies such as chasteberry (Vitex agnus-castus), evening primrose oil, and ginger may offer relief from PMS symptoms by modulating hormonal activity, reducing inflammation, and supporting hormonal balance. These herbs can be taken orally or used topically as part of a holistic approach to managing menstrual health.

Empowering Menstrual Health

Education and Awareness: Empowering women with knowledge about menstrual health and PMS is essential for promoting well-being and reducing stigma surrounding menstruation. By fostering open conversations, providing accurate information, and raising awareness about menstrual health, we can empower women to take charge of their reproductive health and seek support when needed.

Holistic Care: Holistic care approaches menstrual health and PMS from a comprehensive perspective, addressing the physical, emotional, and spiritual aspects of well-being. Integrative therapies such as acupuncture, massage, aromatherapy, and mindfulness practices can complement conventional treatments and offer additional support for managing menstrual health and PMS.

Menstrual health and PMS are integral aspects of women's well-being, reflecting the intricate interplay of hormones, emotions, and physical health throughout the menstrual cycle. By embracing a holistic approach that honors the cyclical nature of menstruation and supports women's unique needs, we can nurture wellness, resilience, and vitality across all phases of the menstrual cycle. Through education, awareness, and compassionate care, we can empower women to embrace their menstrual health journey with confidence, grace, and resilience.

Chaste Tree Berry: Balancing Hormones for Women's Wellness

Introduction

In the realm of herbal medicine, the chaste tree berry, also known as Vitex agnus-castus or simply Vitex, emerges as a powerful ally for women's hormonal health and well-being. With a rich history dating back to ancient times, chaste tree berry has been revered for its ability to balance hormones, regulate menstrual cycles, and alleviate a variety of gynecological concerns. In this chapter, we explore the remarkable properties of chaste tree berry and its role in promoting women's wellness.

Understanding Chaste Tree Berry

Botanical Background: Chaste tree berry is a small, brownish-black fruit that grows on the chaste tree, a shrub native to the Mediterranean region and parts of Asia. The plant belongs to the Verbena family (Verbenaceae) and has a long history of use in traditional herbal medicine, particularly in Greek, Roman, and Ayurvedic traditions. Chaste tree berry is renowned for its hormonal-regulating properties and has been used for centuries to support women's reproductive health.

Medicinal Properties: Chaste tree berry contains a variety of bioactive compounds, including flavonoids, iridoid glycosides, and diterpenes, which contribute to its hormonal-balancing and anti-inflammatory effects. The herb acts on the pituitary gland, helping to regulate the production of hormones such as prolactin, luteinizing hormone (LH), and follicle-stimulating hormone (FSH), which play key roles in menstrual cycle regulation and ovulation.

Harnessing the Power of Chaste Tree Berry

Menstrual Health: Chaste tree berry is best known for its ability to regulate menstrual cycles and alleviate symptoms of hormonal imbalance, such as irregular periods, heavy bleeding, and menstrual cramps. By balancing hormone levels and supporting normal ovulation, chaste tree berry helps restore harmony to the menstrual cycle, promoting regularity and reducing symptoms of discomfort.

Premenstrual Syndrome (PMS): Chaste tree berry may help alleviate symptoms of premenstrual syndrome (PMS), such as mood swings, irritability, breast tenderness, and bloating. The herb's hormone-balancing effects help reduce fluctuations in estrogen and progesterone levels, leading to improved mood, reduced fluid retention, and overall symptom relief.

Menopausal Support: Chaste tree berry may also offer support for women experiencing menopausal symptoms, such as hot flashes, night sweats, and mood changes. By modulating hormone levels and supporting hormonal balance, chaste tree berry can help ease the transition through menopause and alleviate symptoms associated with hormonal fluctuations.

How to Use Chaste Tree Berry

Herbal Supplements: Chaste tree berry supplements are available in various forms, including capsules, tablets, tinctures, and teas. Follow the manufacturer's dosage recommendations for optimal results. Chaste tree berry supplements are typically taken daily for several months to experience the full benefits of hormonal balance and menstrual cycle regulation.

Tinctures and Extracts: Chaste tree berry tinctures or liquid extracts can be added to water or juice and consumed orally for a concentrated dose of therapeutic compounds. Tinctures provide a convenient and potent way to experience the benefits of chaste tree berry, particularly for individuals who prefer liquid formulations.

Teas: Chaste tree berry teas can be brewed using dried chaste tree berries or commercially available tea bags. Steep the berries in hot water for 5-10 minutes, then strain and enjoy the tea warm or chilled. Chaste tree berry tea can be consumed regularly as part of a hormone-balancing regimen for menstrual health and well-being.

Safety Considerations

Chaste tree berry is generally safe for most people when used appropriately. However, it may interact with certain medications, including hormone therapy, birth control pills, and dopamine agonists. Pregnant or breastfeeding women, as well as individuals with hormone-sensitive conditions or certain medical conditions, should consult with a healthcare professional before using chaste tree berry supplements.

Chaste tree berry, with its hormone-balancing properties and centuries-old legacy in women's health, offers a natural solution for menstrual irregularities, PMS symptoms, and menopausal discomfort. By harnessing the power of this remarkable herb, women can restore harmony to their hormonal balance, regulate menstrual cycles, and experience greater well-being throughout all stages of life. With chaste tree berry as a trusted ally in the journey toward hormonal health and vitality, women can embrace their feminine wellness with confidence, resilience, and grace.

Dong Quai: Nurturing Women's Vitality and Hormonal Balance

Introduction

In the realm of traditional Chinese medicine, few herbs hold as revered a status as Dong Quai, also known as Angelica sinensis. Celebrated for its profound effects on women's health and vitality, Dong Quai has been cherished for centuries as a tonic for the female reproductive system. In this chapter, we delve into the rich history, medicinal properties, and therapeutic uses of Dong Quai, shedding light on its role in nurturing women's vitality and hormonal balance.

Understanding Dong Quai

Botanical Background: Dong Quai is a perennial plant native to China, Japan, and Korea, where it has been cultivated and used for medicinal purposes for thousands of years. Belonging to the Umbelliferae family, Dong Quai is characterized by its aromatic roots, hollow stems, and clusters of small white or pink flowers. The root of the Dong Quai plant is the most commonly used part in herbal medicine and is prized for its hormone-balancing and tonic properties.

Medicinal Properties: Dong Quai contains a variety of bioactive compounds, including coumarins, flavonoids, and polysaccharides, which contribute to its hormonal-regulating, anti-inflammatory, and antioxidant effects. The herb acts on the reproductive system, helping to regulate menstrual cycles, alleviate menstrual cramps, and promote overall hormonal balance in women.

Harnessing the Power of Dong Quai

Menstrual Health: Dong Quai is best known for its ability to regulate menstrual cycles and alleviate symptoms of menstrual irregularities, such as irregular periods, painful cramps, and heavy bleeding. The herb's hormone-balancing effects help support normal estrogen levels, promote uterine tone, and reduce muscle spasms, leading to improved menstrual regularity and comfort.

Menopausal Support: Dong Quai may also offer support for women experiencing symptoms of menopause, such as hot flashes, night sweats, and mood changes. By modulating hormone levels and supporting adrenal function, Dong Quai can help ease the transition through menopause and alleviate symptoms associated with hormonal fluctuations.

Reproductive Tonic: Dong Quai is often referred to as a reproductive tonic for women, nourishing the female reproductive system and promoting overall vitality and well-being. The herb's adaptogenic properties help strengthen the body's resilience to stress, support adrenal health, and enhance vitality and energy levels, particularly during times of hormonal imbalance or transition.

How to Use Dong Quai

Herbal Supplements: Dong Quai supplements are available in various forms, including capsules, tablets, tinctures, and teas. Follow the manufacturer's dosage recommendations for optimal results. Dong Quai supplements are typically taken daily for several months to experience the full benefits of hormonal balance and reproductive support.

Tinctures and Extracts: Dong Quai tinctures or liquid extracts can be added to water or juice and consumed orally for a concentrated dose of therapeutic compounds. Tinctures provide a convenient and potent way to experience the benefits of Dong Quai, particularly for individuals who prefer liquid formulations.

Teas: Dong Quai teas can be brewed using dried Dong Quai root or commercially available tea bags. Steep the root in hot water for 5-10 minutes, then strain and enjoy the tea warm or chilled. Dong Quai tea can be consumed regularly as part of a hormone-balancing regimen for menstrual health and well-being.

Safety Considerations

Dong Quai is generally safe for most people when used appropriately. However, it may interact with certain medications, including blood thinners, hormone therapy, and medications metabolized by the liver. Pregnant or breastfeeding women, as well as individuals with hormone-sensitive conditions or certain medical conditions, should consult with a healthcare professional before using Dong Quai supplements.

Dong Quai, with its centuries-old legacy in traditional Chinese medicine and profound effects on women's health and vitality, offers a natural solution for menstrual irregularities, menopausal symptoms, and reproductive health concerns. By harnessing the power of this remarkable herb, women can restore balance to their hormonal system, alleviate discomfort, and enhance vitality and well-being. With Dong Quai as a trusted ally in the journey toward women's wellness, individuals can embrace their feminine vitality with confidence, resilience, and grace.

Raspberry Leaf: Nurturing Women's Wellness from Within

Introduction

Nestled amidst lush green foliage and delicate pink blooms, the raspberry plant harbors a secret treasure within its leaves – a gift to women seeking vitality and wellness throughout life's journey. Raspberry leaf, revered for centuries for its myriad health benefits, holds a special place in herbal medicine as a tonic for the female reproductive system. In this chapter, we explore the enchanting properties of raspberry leaf and its role in nurturing women's wellness from within.

Understanding Raspberry Leaf

Botanical Background: Raspberry leaf, derived from the leaves of the red raspberry plant (Rubus idaeus), is a perennial herb native to Europe, Asia, and North America. Belonging to the Rosaceae family, raspberry plants are characterized by their thorny stems, serrated leaves, and sweet-tart berries. Raspberry leaf has a long history of use in traditional herbal medicine, particularly among indigenous cultures, where it was prized for its tonic and healing properties.

Medicinal Properties: Raspberry leaf contains a wealth of nutrients and bioactive compounds, including vitamins, minerals, tannins, and flavonoids, which contribute to its nourishing, tonifying, and astringent effects on the body. The herb acts on the uterus and reproductive organs, helping to tone the muscles, regulate menstrual cycles, and support overall reproductive health in women.

Harnessing the Power of Raspberry Leaf

Menstrual Health: Raspberry leaf is renowned for its ability to tone the uterus and regulate menstrual cycles, making it a valuable remedy for women experiencing menstrual irregularities, such as irregular periods, heavy bleeding, and painful cramps. The herb's uterine toning properties help strengthen the muscles of the uterus, leading to more regular and comfortable menstrual cycles.

Pregnancy Support: Raspberry leaf is often used during pregnancy to prepare the uterus for childbirth and promote overall pregnancy wellness. The herb's uterine toning effects can help strengthen the uterine muscles, improve circulation to the reproductive organs, and support the body's natural processes during labor and delivery. Raspberry leaf is typically consumed in the third trimester of pregnancy under the guidance of a qualified healthcare provider.

Postpartum Recovery: Raspberry leaf can also be beneficial during the postpartum period, helping to tone the uterus, reduce bleeding, and promote healing after childbirth. The herb's astringent properties help tighten and tone the uterine muscles, supporting the body's recovery process and aiding in the restoration of uterine health and function.

How to Use Raspberry Leaf

Herbal Teas: Raspberry leaf tea is a popular and convenient way to enjoy the benefits of this nourishing herb. Simply steep dried raspberry leaves in hot water for 5-10 minutes, then strain and enjoy the tea warm or chilled. Raspberry leaf tea can be consumed regularly throughout the menstrual cycle or pregnancy to support women's wellness and reproductive health.

Tinctures and Extracts: Raspberry leaf tinctures or liquid extracts can be added to water or juice and consumed orally for a concentrated dose of therapeutic compounds. Tinctures provide a convenient and potent way to experience the benefits of raspberry leaf, particularly for individuals who prefer liquid formulations.

Capsules and Tablets: Raspberry leaf supplements are available in capsule or tablet form for those who prefer a convenient and standardized dosage. Follow the manufacturer's dosage recommendations for optimal results. Raspberry leaf supplements can be taken daily as part of a holistic approach to women's wellness and reproductive health.

Safety Considerations

Raspberry leaf is generally safe for most people when used appropriately. However, pregnant women should consult with a qualified healthcare provider before using raspberry leaf supplements, particularly during the first and second trimesters of pregnancy. Individuals with certain medical conditions or allergies should also exercise caution and seek guidance from a healthcare professional before using raspberry leaf products.

Raspberry leaf, with its nourishing, tonifying, and healing properties, offers a natural and gentle way to support women's wellness and reproductive health throughout life's journey. Whether used to regulate menstrual cycles, prepare for childbirth, or aid in postpartum recovery, raspberry leaf stands as a testament to the wisdom of nature and the power of herbal medicine to nurture and sustain women's vitality from within. With raspberry leaf as a trusted ally in the quest for wellness and balance, women can embrace their feminine health with grace, resilience, and vitality.

Menopause Relief: Embracing Change with Grace and Vitality

Introduction

Menopause marks a profound transition in a woman's life, signaling the end of one chapter and the beginning of another. Yet, amidst the physical changes and hormonal fluctuations that accompany this natural stage of life, menopause also offers an opportunity for renewal, growth, and self-discovery. In this chapter, we explore strategies for finding relief from menopausal symptoms and embracing this transformative journey with grace and vitality.

Understanding Menopause

The Menopausal Transition: Menopause is a natural biological process that typically occurs in women between the ages of 45 and 55, although the timing can vary widely from person to person. It marks the end of menstruation and fertility, signaling the cessation of ovarian function and the decline in hormone production, particularly estrogen and progesterone.

Symptoms of Menopause: Menopause is often accompanied by a range of symptoms, including hot flashes, night sweats, mood swings, vaginal dryness, insomnia, and fatigue. These symptoms can vary in severity and duration, impacting women's quality of life and overall well-being during the menopausal transition.

Finding Relief from Menopausal Symptoms

Hormone Replacement Therapy (HRT): Hormone replacement therapy involves the use of estrogen or estrogen-progestin combinations to alleviate menopausal symptoms, such as hot flashes, vaginal dryness, and mood swings. HRT can be administered in various forms, including pills, patches, creams, and vaginal rings, and is available in different dosages to meet individual needs.

Natural Remedies: Several natural remedies and lifestyle modifications may help alleviate menopausal symptoms and support overall well-being during this transition. These include:

- Herbal Supplements: Certain herbs, such as black cohosh, red clover, and soy isoflavones, have been traditionally used to alleviate menopausal symptoms. These herbs may help regulate hormone levels, reduce hot flashes, and improve mood and sleep quality.

- Dietary Changes: A balanced diet rich in fruits, vegetables, whole grains, and healthy fats can support hormonal balance and overall well-being during menopause. Limiting caffeine, alcohol, and spicy foods may help reduce hot flashes and night sweats.

- Regular Exercise: Engaging in regular physical activity, such as walking, swimming, or yoga, can help relieve stress, improve mood, and promote overall health and vitality during menopause.

- Stress Management: Practicing stress-reduction techniques, such as deep breathing, meditation, or mindfulness, can help alleviate menopausal symptoms and improve overall quality of life.

- Supplements: Certain vitamins and minerals, such as calcium, vitamin D, and magnesium, may help support bone health and reduce the risk of osteoporosis during menopause. Omega-3 fatty acids may also help alleviate symptoms of depression and mood swings.

Alternative Therapies: Acupuncture, chiropractic care, massage therapy, and other alternative therapies may offer relief from menopausal symptoms by promoting relaxation, reducing stress, and restoring balance to the body's energy systems.

Embracing Menopause with Grace and Vitality

Self-Care Practices: Embracing self-care practices can help women navigate the physical and emotional changes of menopause with grace and vitality. This may include:

- Self-Compassion: Practicing self-compassion and self-acceptance can help women embrace their changing bodies and identities with grace and resilience.

- Connection: Maintaining social connections and seeking support from friends, family, or support groups can help women feel less isolated and more empowered during the menopausal transition.

- Creativity: Exploring creative outlets, such as art, writing, or music, can provide a sense of fulfillment and purpose during this transformative time.

- Mindfulness: Cultivating mindfulness and present-moment awareness can help women navigate the ups and downs of menopause with greater ease and acceptance.

Professional Support: Seeking support from healthcare providers, counselors, or menopause specialists can provide women with personalized guidance, education, and treatment options to address their specific needs and concerns during menopause.

Menopause, though often accompanied by physical and emotional challenges, also offers an opportunity for growth, renewal, and self-discovery. By embracing natural remedies, self-care practices, and professional support, women can find relief from menopausal symptoms and navigate this transformative journey with grace, resilience, and vitality. With a holistic approach to menopause relief, women can embrace this new chapter of life with open hearts and empowered spirits, embracing change as an opportunity for growth, wisdom, and renewal.

Black Cohosh: Empowering Women's Wellness Through Menopause

Introduction

Amidst the gentle sway of forest canopies, the black cohosh plant stands tall, its graceful white flowers and dark, knotted roots concealing a treasure trove of healing properties. For generations, indigenous cultures revered black cohosh as a sacred remedy for women's health, particularly during the transformative stages of menopause. In this chapter, we unravel the mysteries of black cohosh and explore its empowering role in supporting women's wellness through the journey of menopause.

Understanding Black Cohosh

Botanical Background: Black cohosh, scientifically known as Actaea racemosa or Cimicifuga racemosa, is a perennial herb native to North America, where it thrives in the cool, shaded woodlands of the eastern United States and Canada. The plant belongs to the Ranunculaceae family and is distinguished by its tall, slender stems, feathery compound leaves, and spiky clusters of small white flowers. The roots of the black cohosh plant are the most commonly used part in herbal medicine and contain the plant's potent medicinal compounds.

Medicinal Properties: Black cohosh contains a variety of bioactive compounds, including triterpene glycosides, phenolic acids, and alkaloids, which contribute to its hormone-regulating, anti-inflammatory, and analgesic effects. The herb acts on the endocrine system, particularly the hypothalamus and pituitary gland, helping to modulate hormone levels and alleviate symptoms associated with hormonal imbalance, such as hot flashes, night sweats, mood swings, and vaginal dryness.

Harnessing the Power of Black Cohosh

Menopausal Symptom Relief: Black cohosh is best known for its ability to alleviate symptoms of menopause, making it a popular remedy for women seeking relief from hot flashes, night sweats, and other discomforts associated with hormonal fluctuations. The herb's hormone-regulating effects help balance estrogen levels and modulate neurotransmitter activity in the brain, leading to reduced frequency and severity of menopausal symptoms.

Bone Health: Black cohosh may also offer support for bone health during menopause, helping to reduce the risk of osteoporosis and bone fractures. The herb's estrogen-like effects help maintain bone density and prevent bone loss associated with hormonal changes during menopause.

Mood and Emotional Well-being: Black cohosh has been traditionally used to support mood and emotional well-being during menopause, helping to reduce irritability, anxiety, and depression associated with hormonal fluctuations. The herb's calming and mood-stabilizing effects can promote a sense of emotional balance and resilience during this transitional phase of life.

How to Use Black Cohosh

Herbal Supplements: Black cohosh supplements are available in various forms, including capsules, tablets, tinctures, and teas. Follow the manufacturer's dosage recommendations for optimal results. Black cohosh supplements are typically taken daily for several weeks to experience the full benefits of hormonal balance and symptom relief.

Tinctures and Extracts: Black cohosh tinctures or liquid extracts can be added to water or juice and consumed orally for a concentrated dose of therapeutic compounds. Tinctures provide a convenient and potent way to experience the benefits of black cohosh, particularly for individuals who prefer liquid formulations.

Teas: Black cohosh teas can be brewed using dried black cohosh root or commercially available tea bags. Steep the root in hot water for 5-10 minutes, then strain and enjoy the tea warm or chilled. Black cohosh tea can be consumed regularly as part of a hormone-balancing regimen for menopausal symptom relief.

Safety Considerations

Black cohosh is generally safe for most people when used appropriately. However, it may interact with certain medications, including hormone therapy, blood thinners, and medications metabolized by the liver. Pregnant or breastfeeding women, as well as individuals with certain medical conditions or allergies, should consult with a healthcare professional before using black cohosh supplements.

Black cohosh, with its potent medicinal properties and time-honored legacy in women's health, offers a natural and empowering solution for menopausal symptom relief. By harnessing the power of this remarkable herb, women can find relief from hot flashes, night sweats, and other discomforts associated with menopause, reclaiming their vitality and well-being during this transformative phase of life. With black cohosh as a trusted ally in the journey toward hormonal balance and empowerment, women can embrace the menopausal transition with grace, resilience, and vitality, stepping confidently into the next chapter of their lives with renewed strength and vitality.

Red Clover: Nature's Nourishment for Women's Wellness

Introduction

In the meadows and fields, where the sun kisses the earth and wildflowers dance in the breeze, the humble red clover graces the landscape with its vibrant blooms and delicate foliage. Yet, beyond its picturesque appearance, red clover harbors a secret treasure – a bounty of healing compounds that have been cherished for centuries for their profound effects on women's health and well-being. In this chapter, we embark on a journey to explore the enchanting properties of red clover and its role in nurturing women's wellness.

Understanding Red Clover

Botanical Background: Red clover, scientifically known as Trifolium pratense, is a perennial legume native to Europe, Asia, and North Africa, where it thrives in meadows, grasslands, and agricultural fields. The plant belongs to the Fabaceae family and is characterized by its distinctive three-lobed leaves, clusters of pink to purple flowers, and long, slender stems. Red clover has a long history of use in traditional herbal medicine, particularly among indigenous cultures, where it was revered for its medicinal properties.

Medicinal Properties: Red clover contains a variety of bioactive compounds, including isoflavones, flavonoids, and phytoestrogens, which contribute to its hormone-balancing, anti-inflammatory, and antioxidant effects. The herb acts on the endocrine system, particularly the estrogen receptors, helping to regulate hormone levels and alleviate symptoms associated with hormonal imbalance, such as hot flashes, night sweats, mood swings, and vaginal dryness.

Harnessing the Power of Red Clover

Menopausal Symptom Relief: Red clover is best known for its ability to alleviate symptoms of menopause, making it a popular remedy for women seeking relief from hot flashes, night sweats, and other discomforts associated with hormonal fluctuations. The herb's estrogen-like effects help balance hormone levels and modulate neurotransmitter activity in the brain, leading to reduced frequency and severity of menopausal symptoms.

Bone Health: Red clover may also offer support for bone health during menopause, helping to reduce the risk of osteoporosis and bone fractures. The herb's isoflavones have been shown to promote bone density and inhibit bone loss associated with hormonal changes during menopause.

Heart Health: Red clover has been traditionally used to support heart health and reduce the risk of cardiovascular disease. The herb's antioxidant and anti-inflammatory properties help protect against oxidative stress and inflammation in the blood vessels, promoting healthy circulation and cardiovascular function.

How to Use Red Clover

Herbal Supplements: Red clover supplements are available in various forms, including capsules, tablets, tinctures, and teas. Follow the manufacturer's dosage recommendations for optimal results. Red clover supplements are typically taken daily for several weeks to experience the full benefits of hormonal balance and symptom relief.

Tinctures and Extracts: Red clover tinctures or liquid extracts can be added to water or juice and consumed orally for a concentrated dose of therapeutic compounds. Tinctures provide a convenient and potent way to experience the benefits of red clover, particularly for individuals who prefer liquid formulations.

Teas: Red clover teas can be brewed using dried red clover flowers or commercially available tea bags. Steep the flowers in hot water for 5-10 minutes, then strain and enjoy the tea warm or chilled. Red clover tea can be consumed regularly as part of a hormone-balancing regimen for menopausal symptom relief.

Safety Considerations

Red clover is generally safe for most people when used appropriately. However, it may interact with certain medications, including hormone therapy, blood thinners, and medications metabolized by the liver. Pregnant or breastfeeding women, as well as individuals with certain medical conditions or allergies, should consult with a healthcare professional before using red clover supplements.

Red clover, with its potent medicinal properties and time-honored legacy in women's health, offers a natural and nurturing solution for menopausal symptom relief. By harnessing the power of this remarkable herb, women can find relief from hot flashes, night sweats, and other discomforts associated with menopause, reclaiming their vitality and well-being during this transformative phase of life. With red clover as a trusted ally in the journey toward hormonal balance and empowerment, women can embrace the menopausal transition with grace, resilience, and vitality, stepping confidently into the next chapter of their lives with renewed strength and vitality.

Sage: Wisdom from Nature for Women's Health

Introduction

In the sun-drenched hillsides and rocky cliffs, where the earth meets the sky in a harmonious embrace, sage flourishes, its silvery leaves and delicate blooms whispering ancient wisdom to those who listen. For millennia, sage has been revered for its myriad healing properties, offering solace and support to women as they navigate the ebbs and flows of life. In this chapter, we delve into the profound depths of sage's wisdom and explore its empowering role in women's health and well-being.

Understanding Sage

Botanical Background: Sage, scientifically known as Salvia officinalis, is a perennial herb native to the Mediterranean region, where it thrives in dry, rocky soils and sunny climates. Belonging to the Lamiaceae family, sage is characterized by its aromatic leaves, which are gray-green in color and densely covered with fine hairs. The plant produces clusters of small, purple, blue, or white flowers that bloom in the summer months.

Medicinal Properties: Sage contains a wealth of bioactive compounds, including essential oils, flavonoids, phenolic acids, and rosmarinic acid, which contribute to its anti-inflammatory, antioxidant, antimicrobial, and hormone-regulating effects. The herb acts on the body's systems, particularly the endocrine and nervous systems, helping to modulate hormone levels, reduce inflammation, and support overall health and well-being.

Harnessing the Power of Sage

Menopausal Symptom Relief: Sage is best known for its ability to alleviate symptoms of menopause, making it a popular remedy for women seeking relief from hot flashes, night sweats, and other discomforts associated with hormonal fluctuations. The herb's estrogen-like effects help balance hormone levels and modulate neurotransmitter activity in the brain, leading to reduced frequency and severity of menopausal symptoms.

Memory and Cognitive Function: Sage has been traditionally used to support memory and cognitive function, particularly in older adults. The herb's antioxidant and anti-inflammatory properties help protect brain cells from oxidative stress and inflammation, promoting cognitive health and mental clarity.

Digestive Health: Sage is often used to support digestive health and alleviate symptoms of indigestion, bloating, and gas. The herb's essential oils stimulate digestive enzyme production, improve bile flow, and reduce inflammation in the digestive tract, leading to improved digestion and nutrient absorption.

How to Use Sage

Herbal Supplements: Sage supplements are available in various forms, including capsules, tablets, tinctures, and teas. Follow the manufacturer's dosage recommendations for optimal results. Sage supplements are typically taken daily for several weeks to experience the full benefits of hormonal balance and symptom relief.

Tinctures and Extracts: Sage tinctures or liquid extracts can be added to water or juice and consumed orally for a concentrated dose of therapeutic compounds. Tinctures provide a convenient and potent way to experience the benefits of sage, particularly for individuals who prefer liquid formulations.

Teas: Sage teas can be brewed using dried sage leaves or commercially available tea bags. Steep the leaves in hot water for 5-10 minutes, then strain and enjoy the tea warm or chilled. Sage tea can be consumed regularly as part of a hormone-balancing regimen for menopausal symptom relief.

Safety Considerations

Sage is generally safe for most people when used appropriately. However, it may interact with certain medications, including hormone therapy, blood thinners, and medications metabolized by the liver. Pregnant or breastfeeding women, as well as individuals with certain medical conditions or allergies, should consult with a healthcare professional before using sage supplements.

Sage, with its potent medicinal properties and timeless wisdom, offers a natural and empowering solution for women's health and well-being. By harnessing the power of this remarkable herb, women can find relief from menopausal symptoms, support cognitive function, and promote digestive health, reclaiming their vitality and strength as they embrace the journey of life with grace and wisdom. With sage as a trusted ally in the quest for holistic wellness, women can cultivate resilience, balance, and harmony in body, mind, and spirit, honoring the wisdom of nature and the inherent healing power within.

Wild Yam: Nurturing Women's Wellness Naturally

Introduction

In the heart of dense forests and along the banks of winding rivers, the wild yam vine unfurls its vibrant foliage, offering a verdant haven for creatures great and small. Yet, beneath its lush canopy lies a hidden treasure – the humble wild yam root, revered for centuries for its profound healing properties. In this chapter, we embark on a journey to uncover the remarkable benefits of wild yam and its nurturing role in women's health and wellness.

Understanding Wild Yam

Botanical Background: Wild yam, scientifically known as Dioscorea villosa, is a perennial vine native to North and Central America, where it thrives in rich, moist soils and shaded woodlands. Belonging to the Dioscoreaceae family, wild yam is characterized by its twining stems, heart-shaped leaves, and clusters of small, greenish-yellow flowers. The plant produces knobby, tuberous roots that have been prized for their medicinal properties since ancient times.

Medicinal Properties: Wild yam contains a variety of bioactive compounds, including diosgenin, saponins, and phytosterols, which contribute to its hormone-balancing, anti-inflammatory, and antispasmodic effects. The herb acts on the endocrine system, particularly the adrenal glands and ovaries, helping to regulate hormone levels and alleviate symptoms associated with hormonal imbalance, such as hot flashes, night sweats, mood swings, and menstrual irregularities.

Harnessing the Power of Wild Yam

Hormone Balance: Wild yam is best known for its ability to support hormone balance, making it a popular remedy for women seeking relief from menopausal symptoms, PMS, and menstrual irregularities. The herb's diosgenin content serves as a precursor to progesterone, a key hormone involved in regulating the menstrual cycle and supporting reproductive health.

Menopausal Symptom Relief: Wild yam may help alleviate symptoms of menopause, such as hot flashes, night sweats, and mood swings, by supporting hormone balance and reducing the frequency and severity of hormonal fluctuations.

Reproductive Health: Wild yam has been traditionally used to support reproductive health and fertility in women. The herb's hormone-balancing effects may help regulate menstrual cycles, improve ovulation, and enhance fertility in women experiencing hormonal imbalances or menstrual irregularities.

How to Use Wild Yam

Herbal Supplements: Wild yam supplements are available in various forms, including capsules, tablets, tinctures, and creams. Follow the manufacturer's dosage recommendations for optimal results. Wild yam supplements are typically taken daily for several weeks to experience the full benefits of hormonal balance and symptom relief.

Topical Creams: Wild yam creams or ointments can be applied topically to the skin for localized relief of menopausal symptoms, such as hot flashes and vaginal dryness. Massage a small amount of wild yam cream onto the skin as needed, focusing on areas of discomfort or irritation.

Safety Considerations

Wild yam is generally safe for most people when used appropriately. However, it may interact with certain medications, including hormone therapy, blood thinners, and medications metabolized by the liver. Pregnant or breastfeeding women, as well as individuals with certain medical conditions or allergies, should consult with a healthcare professional before using wild yam supplements.

Wild yam, with its potent medicinal properties and time-honored legacy in women's health, offers a natural and nurturing solution for hormone balance and reproductive wellness. By harnessing the power of this remarkable herb, women can find relief from menopausal symptoms, support menstrual health, and enhance fertility, reclaiming their vitality and well-being as they embrace the journey of womanhood with grace and resilience. With wild yam as a trusted ally in the quest for holistic wellness, women can cultivate balance, harmony, and vitality in body, mind, and spirit, honoring the wisdom of nature and the inherent healing power within.

Reproductive Health: Nurturing the Sacred Cycle of Life

Introduction

In the intricate tapestry of life, the cycle of reproduction weaves a thread of continuity, perpetuating the miracle of existence from one generation to the next. Yet, within this sacred journey, women bear the unique responsibility of nurturing and safeguarding the gift of life within their bodies. In this chapter, we embark on a journey to explore the intricate workings of reproductive health, delving into the multifaceted aspects of fertility, menstruation, and hormonal balance, and uncovering the natural remedies and holistic practices that support women's well-being throughout the reproductive cycle.

Understanding Reproductive Health

Fertility and Conception: Fertility, the ability to conceive and bear offspring, is a central aspect of reproductive health. It relies on a delicate interplay of hormones, ovarian function, and reproductive anatomy, culminating in the release of a mature egg from the ovary and its subsequent fertilization by sperm. Factors such as age, hormonal balance, lifestyle choices, and underlying health conditions can influence fertility and reproductive outcomes.

Menstrual Health: Menstruation, or the monthly shedding of the uterine lining, is a natural and integral part of the reproductive cycle in women of reproductive age. It is governed by complex hormonal fluctuations, particularly estrogen and progesterone, which regulate the growth and shedding of the uterine lining. Menstrual health encompasses various aspects, including the regularity and duration of menstrual cycles, the presence of menstrual symptoms, and the overall impact on physical and emotional well-being.

Hormonal Balance: Hormonal balance plays a crucial role in reproductive health, influencing menstrual regularity, ovulation, and fertility. Hormones such as estrogen, progesterone, luteinizing hormone (LH), and follicle-stimulating hormone (FSH) orchestrate the intricate dance of the menstrual cycle, guiding the development of ovarian follicles, the release of mature eggs, and the preparation of the uterine lining for potential pregnancy. Imbalances in hormone levels can disrupt the menstrual cycle, leading to irregular periods, anovulation, and fertility challenges.

Supporting Reproductive Health Naturally

Nutrition and Diet: A balanced and nutrient-rich diet forms the foundation of reproductive health, providing essential vitamins, minerals, and antioxidants needed for hormone production, ovarian function, and overall well-being. Foods rich in omega-3 fatty acids, antioxidants, fiber, and plant-based proteins support hormonal balance, reduce inflammation, and promote fertility.

Herbal Remedies: Herbal remedies have been used for centuries to support reproductive health and address various menstrual and fertility concerns. Herbs such as chasteberry (Vitex agnus-castus), red raspberry leaf (Rubus idaeus), dong quai (Angelica sinensis), and maca root (Lepidium meyenii) are commonly used to regulate menstrual cycles, support ovulation, and enhance fertility.

Lifestyle Modifications: Lifestyle factors such as stress, sleep quality, physical activity, and exposure to environmental toxins can profoundly impact reproductive health. Implementing stress-reduction techniques, prioritizing sleep, engaging in regular exercise, and minimizing exposure to endocrine-disrupting chemicals can help support hormonal balance, optimize fertility, and promote overall well-being.

Holistic Practices: Holistic approaches to reproductive health, including acupuncture, chiropractic care, massage therapy, and mind-body therapies, can complement conventional treatments and offer additional support for menstrual irregularities, fertility challenges, and hormonal imbalances.

Reproductive health is a sacred and intricate aspect of women's well-being, encompassing the delicate balance of fertility, menstruation, and hormonal harmony. By nurturing the body, mind, and spirit through wholesome nutrition, herbal remedies, lifestyle modifications, and holistic practices, women can cultivate resilience, balance, and vitality throughout the reproductive cycle. With a holistic approach to reproductive health, women can honor the sacred cycle of life, embrace the gift of fertility, and empower themselves to live in harmony with the natural rhythms of the body, honoring the sacred journey of womanhood with grace, resilience, and vitality.

Maca Root: Nature's Energizing Ally for Hormonal Balance

Introduction

Nestled in the rugged Andean mountains of Peru, amidst the crisp mountain air and fertile soil, thrives a resilient plant with a storied history of nourishing both body and spirit – maca root. Revered for centuries by indigenous cultures for its remarkable health benefits, maca root has gained global acclaim as a natural remedy for hormonal balance, vitality, and overall well-being. In this chapter, we embark on a journey to uncover the secrets of maca root and explore its empowering role in women's health.

Understanding Maca Root

Botanical Background: Maca, scientifically known as Lepidium meyenii, is a hardy biennial plant belonging to the Brassicaceae family. Indigenous to the high-altitude regions of the Andes Mountains in Peru, maca thrives in harsh conditions, where it has been cultivated for thousands of years as a staple food crop and medicinal herb. The plant produces a radish-like root, which varies in color from creamy white to deep purple, and is prized for its adaptogenic properties and nutritional richness.

Medicinal Properties: Maca root is renowned for its unique combination of bioactive compounds, including amino acids, vitamins, minerals, and plant sterols, which contribute to its adaptogenic, hormone-balancing, and energizing effects. The root contains a diverse array of phytonutrients, including macamides and macaenes, which have been shown to support endocrine function, enhance libido, and alleviate symptoms of hormonal imbalance.

Harnessing the Power of Maca Root

Hormonal Balance: Maca root is best known for its ability to support hormonal balance, making it a popular remedy for women seeking relief from menstrual irregularities, menopausal symptoms, and hormonal imbalances. The herb's adaptogenic properties help regulate hormone levels by modulating the hypothalamic-pituitary-adrenal (HPA) axis, leading to improved mood, energy, and overall well-being.

Energy and Vitality: Maca root is prized for its energizing effects, providing a natural boost to physical stamina, endurance, and mental clarity. The root's rich nutrient profile, including carbohydrates, protein, and essential minerals such as calcium, potassium, and iron, supports sustained energy production and enhances vitality and resilience.

Libido and Sexual Health: Maca root has a long history of use as an aphrodisiac and libido enhancer, particularly for women experiencing diminished sexual desire or arousal. The herb's hormone-balancing effects help support sexual function and satisfaction, while its adaptogenic properties reduce stress and anxiety, promoting a healthy and fulfilling sex life.

How to Use Maca Root

Powder: Maca root powder is a versatile and convenient way to incorporate this superfood into your daily routine. Add a spoonful of maca powder to smoothies, yogurt, oatmeal, or baked goods for a nutritious boost of energy and vitality.

Capsules: Maca root capsules provide a convenient and standardized dosage of the herb's active compounds. Take maca capsules with water or your favorite beverage as directed by the manufacturer for optimal results.

Tinctures: Maca root tinctures or liquid extracts offer a concentrated dose of the herb's medicinal compounds. Add a few drops of maca tincture to water or juice and consume orally for quick absorption and maximum potency.

Safety Considerations

Maca root is generally considered safe for most people when consumed in moderate amounts. However, individuals with hormone-sensitive conditions, such as breast cancer, uterine fibroids, or endometriosis, should exercise caution and consult with a healthcare professional before using maca root supplements. Pregnant or breastfeeding women, as well as individuals with certain medical conditions or allergies, should also seek guidance from a qualified healthcare provider before incorporating maca root into their regimen.

Maca root, with its potent medicinal properties and time-honored legacy in women's health, offers a natural and empowering solution for hormonal balance, vitality, and overall well-being. By harnessing the power of this remarkable herb, women can support their reproductive health, enhance their energy and vitality, and reclaim their vitality and resilience. With maca root as a trusted ally in the quest for holistic wellness, women can cultivate balance, harmony, and vitality in body, mind, and spirit, embracing the journey of womanhood with grace, resilience, and vitality.

Shatavari: Nurturing Women's Wellness with Nature's Elixir

Introduction

In the heart of lush Indian forests and verdant valleys, the Shatavari plant unfurls its delicate tendrils, reaching toward the sun with a quiet grace that belies its profound healing properties. Revered for centuries in Ayurvedic medicine as a sacred herb for women's health, Shatavari embodies the essence of feminine vitality and nourishment. In this chapter, we embark on a journey to explore the transformative powers of Shatavari and its nurturing role in women's wellness.

Understanding Shatavari

Botanical Background: Shatavari, scientifically known as Asparagus racemosus, is a perennial climbing vine native to India, Sri Lanka, and other regions of Southeast Asia. Belonging to the Asparagaceae family, Shatavari is characterized by its feathery foliage, slender stems, and fragrant white flowers that bloom in clusters. The plant produces tuberous roots that have been prized for their medicinal properties and culinary uses for thousands of years.

Medicinal Properties: Shatavari is revered for its rich array of bioactive compounds, including saponins, alkaloids, flavonoids, and steroidal glycosides, which contribute to its adaptogenic, hormone-balancing, and rejuvenating effects. The herb acts on the endocrine system, particularly the reproductive organs and adrenal glands, helping to regulate hormone levels, support fertility, and alleviate symptoms of hormonal imbalance.

Harnessing the Power of Shatavari

Hormonal Balance: Shatavari is renowned for its ability to support hormonal balance in women, making it a cherished remedy for menstrual irregularities, menopausal symptoms, and reproductive health concerns. The herb's adaptogenic properties help modulate the hypothalamic-pituitary-adrenal (HPA) axis, leading to improved hormone production, regulation, and overall well-being.

Reproductive Health: Shatavari is prized for its nourishing and tonifying effects on the female reproductive system, promoting fertility, and supporting overall reproductive health. The herb's estrogen-like properties help regulate menstrual cycles, enhance ovarian function, and improve uterine tone, while its adaptogenic properties reduce stress and support emotional well-being.

Digestive Health: Shatavari has been traditionally used to support digestive health and alleviate symptoms of indigestion, acidity, and gastrointestinal discomfort. The herb's demulcent and anti-inflammatory properties soothe and protect the digestive tract, promoting healthy digestion and nutrient absorption.

How to Use Shatavari

Powder: Shatavari powder is a versatile and convenient way to incorporate this nourishing herb into your daily routine. Add a spoonful of Shatavari powder to smoothies, yogurt, oatmeal, or warm beverages for a nourishing boost of vitality and well-being.

Capsules: Shatavari capsules provide a standardized dosage of the herb's active compounds, making them a convenient option for daily supplementation. Take Shatavari capsules with water or your favorite beverage as directed by the manufacturer for optimal results.

Tinctures: Shatavari tinctures or liquid extracts offer a concentrated dose of the herb's medicinal compounds. Add a few drops of Shatavari tincture to water or juice and consume orally for quick absorption and maximum potency.

Safety Considerations

Shatavari is generally considered safe for most people when consumed in moderate amounts. However, individuals with hormone-sensitive conditions, such as breast cancer, uterine fibroids, or endometriosis, should exercise caution and consult with a healthcare professional before using Shatavari supplements. Pregnant or breastfeeding women, as well as individuals with certain medical conditions or allergies, should also seek guidance from a qualified healthcare provider before incorporating Shatavari into their regimen.

Shatavari, with its potent medicinal properties and time-honored legacy in women's health, offers a natural and nurturing solution for hormonal balance, fertility, and overall well-being. By harnessing the power of this remarkable herb, women can support their reproductive health, enhance their vitality, and reclaim their strength and resilience. With Shatavari as a trusted ally in the quest for holistic wellness, women can cultivate balance, harmony, and vitality in body, mind, and spirit, embracing the journey of womanhood with grace, resilience, and vitality.

Vitex: Restoring Hormonal Harmony for Women's Wellness

Introduction

Amidst the tranquil landscapes of the Mediterranean region, the Vitex plant stands as a beacon of hope for women seeking balance and harmony within their bodies. With its delicate blooms and aromatic foliage, Vitex has long been revered for its profound influence on hormonal health and overall well-being. In this chapter, we embark on a journey to explore the healing virtues of Vitex and its transformative role in restoring hormonal harmony for women's wellness.

Understanding Vitex

Botanical Background: Vitex, scientifically known as Vitex agnus-castus, is a deciduous shrub native to the Mediterranean region and parts of Asia. Belonging to the Verbenaceae family, Vitex is characterized by its palmate leaves, clusters of small lavender-blue flowers, and dark purple berries. The plant has a rich history of use in traditional herbal medicine, particularly in ancient Greece and Rome, where it was prized for its medicinal properties and symbolic significance.

Medicinal Properties: Vitex is renowned for its ability to influence hormonal balance and regulate the menstrual cycle, making it a cherished remedy for women's health concerns. The herb contains a variety of bioactive compounds, including flavonoids, iridoid glycosides, and essential oils, which act on the hypothalamus and pituitary glands to modulate hormone levels and support reproductive function.

Harnessing the Power of Vitex

Hormonal Balance: Vitex is best known for its hormone-regulating effects, particularly its ability to balance levels of estrogen and progesterone in the body. The herb's action on the hypothalamic-pituitary axis helps regulate the production of luteinizing hormone (LH) and follicle-stimulating hormone (FSH), leading to improved hormonal balance and menstrual regularity.

Menstrual Health: Vitex is prized for its ability to alleviate symptoms of menstrual irregularities, such as irregular cycles, PMS, and menstrual cramps. The herb's hormone-balancing effects help regulate the menstrual cycle, reduce menstrual pain and discomfort, and promote overall menstrual health and well-being.

Fertility Support: Vitex is commonly used to support fertility and enhance reproductive health in women. The herb's ability to regulate hormone levels and promote ovulation can improve fertility outcomes and increase the chances of conception for women struggling with infertility or subfertility.

How to Use Vitex

Tinctures: Vitex tinctures or liquid extracts offer a concentrated dose of the herb's medicinal compounds. Add a few drops of Vitex tincture to water or juice and consume orally for quick absorption and maximum potency.

Capsules: Vitex capsules provide a standardized dosage of the herb's active compounds, making them a convenient option for daily supplementation. Take Vitex capsules with water or your favorite beverage as directed by the manufacturer for optimal results.

Teas: Vitex teas can be brewed using dried Vitex berries or commercially available tea bags. Steep the berries or tea bags in hot water for 5-10 minutes, then strain and enjoy the tea warm or chilled. Vitex tea can be consumed regularly as part of a hormone-balancing regimen for women's health.

Safety Considerations

Vitex is generally considered safe for most people when used appropriately. However, it may interact with certain medications, including hormonal contraceptives, hormone replacement therapy, and dopamine-related medications. Pregnant or breastfeeding women, as well as individuals with certain medical conditions or allergies, should consult with a healthcare professional before using Vitex supplements.

Vitex, with its potent medicinal properties and time-honored legacy in women's health, offers a natural and empowering solution for hormonal balance, menstrual health, and fertility support. By harnessing the power of this remarkable herb, women can restore harmony and vitality within their bodies, reclaiming their health and well-being with grace and resilience. With Vitex as a trusted ally in the quest for holistic wellness, women can cultivate balance, harmony, and vitality in body, mind, and spirit, embracing the journey of womanhood with grace, resilience, and vitality.

Tribulus: Unleashing Vitality and Strength for Women's Wellness

Introduction

Nestled in the sun-kissed landscapes of Eastern Europe, Asia, and Africa, the Tribulus plant emerges as a symbol of resilience and vitality, offering a potent elixir for women seeking to unleash their inner strength and vitality. Revered for centuries in traditional herbal medicine for its transformative effects on hormonal balance and reproductive health, Tribulus stands as a beacon of hope for women embarking on their wellness journey. In this chapter, we delve into the remarkable virtues of Tribulus and its empowering role in enhancing women's vitality and well-being.

Understanding Tribulus

Botanical Background: Tribulus, scientifically known as Tribulus terrestris, is a flowering plant belonging to the Zygophyllaceae family. Indigenous to warm temperate and tropical regions, Tribulus is characterized by its low-growing stature, spiny leaves, and vibrant yellow flowers that bloom in clusters. The plant produces small, spiny fruits containing seeds that have been used for centuries in traditional herbal medicine for their medicinal properties.

Medicinal Properties: Tribulus is renowned for its rich array of bioactive compounds, including saponins, flavonoids, alkaloids, and steroidal glycosides, which contribute to its adaptogenic, hormone-balancing, and rejuvenating effects. The herb acts on the endocrine system, particularly the reproductive organs and adrenal glands, helping to regulate hormone levels, support fertility, and enhance overall vitality and well-being.

Harnessing the Power of Tribulus

Hormonal Balance: Tribulus is best known for its ability to support hormonal balance in women, making it a cherished remedy for menstrual irregularities, menopausal symptoms, and reproductive health concerns. The herb's adaptogenic properties help modulate the hypothalamic-pituitary-adrenal (HPA) axis, leading to improved hormone production, regulation, and overall well-being.

Fertility Support: Tribulus is commonly used to support fertility and enhance reproductive health in women. The herb's ability to regulate hormone levels and promote ovulation can improve fertility outcomes and increase the chances of conception for women struggling with infertility or subfertility.

Physical Endurance: Tribulus is prized for its energizing effects and ability to enhance physical endurance, stamina, and athletic performance. The herb's adaptogenic properties support adrenal function, reduce fatigue, and improve resilience to physical and mental stress, helping women maintain peak performance and vitality.

How to Use Tribulus

Capsules: Tribulus capsules provide a standardized dosage of the herb's active compounds, making them a convenient option for daily supplementation. Take Tribulus capsules with water or your favorite beverage as directed by the manufacturer for optimal results.

Powder: Tribulus powder can be mixed into smoothies, yogurt, oatmeal, or warm beverages for a nourishing boost of vitality and well-being. Add a spoonful of Tribulus powder to your favorite recipes to enjoy its invigorating effects.

Tinctures: Tribulus tinctures or liquid extracts offer a concentrated dose of the herb's medicinal compounds. Add a few drops of Tribulus tincture to water or juice and consume orally for quick absorption and maximum potency.

Safety Considerations

Tribulus is generally considered safe for most people when consumed in moderate amounts. However, individuals with hormone-sensitive conditions, such as breast cancer, uterine fibroids, or endometriosis, should exercise caution and consult with a healthcare professional before using Tribulus supplements. Pregnant or breastfeeding women, as well as individuals with certain medical conditions or allergies, should also seek guidance from a qualified healthcare provider before incorporating Tribulus into their regimen.

Tribulus, with its potent medicinal properties and time-honored legacy in women's health, offers a natural and empowering solution for hormonal balance, fertility support, and overall vitality and well-being. By harnessing the power of this remarkable herb, women can unleash their inner strength, vitality, and resilience, reclaiming their health and vitality with grace and confidence. With Tribulus as a trusted ally in the quest for holistic wellness, women can cultivate balance, harmony, and vitality in body, mind, and spirit, embracing the journey of womanhood with grace, resilience, and vitality.

Nurturing Nature: Exploring Herbs for Children's Health

Introduction

In the gentle embrace of nature's bounty lies a treasure trove of healing wonders, offering solace and support to the most precious among us – our children. From the soothing touch of aloe vera to the comforting warmth of chamomile, herbs have long played a vital role in nurturing the health and well-being of children throughout the ages. In this exploration, we embark on a journey into the enchanting world of herbs for children's health, uncovering the gentle remedies and time-honored traditions that promote vitality, resilience, and joy in our little ones.

Understanding Herbs for Children's Health

Botanical Allies: Herbs have been cherished for their medicinal properties since ancient times, providing natural solutions for a myriad of childhood ailments, from tummy troubles to teething woes. Each herb offers its own unique gifts, whether it's the calming influence of lavender or the immune-boosting power of elderberry, allowing parents to support their children's health holistically and gently.

Gentle Remedies: Unlike harsh chemicals and synthetic compounds, herbs offer a gentle approach to wellness that resonates with the delicate balance of a child's body. Whether administered as teas, tinctures, or herbal baths, these botanical remedies work in harmony with the body's natural rhythms, providing comfort and relief without the risk of harmful side effects.

Cultural Traditions: Across cultures and civilizations, herbal remedies have been passed down through generations, embodying the wisdom and traditions of our ancestors. From Ayurveda to Traditional Chinese Medicine, herbal lore offers a rich tapestry of knowledge and practices that celebrate the interconnectedness of mind, body, and spirit in promoting children's health and vitality.

Exploring the Healing Power of Herbs

Immune Support: Herbs such as echinacea, astragalus, and elderberry offer potent immune-boosting properties, helping to strengthen children's defenses against colds, flu, and other infections. These botanical allies provide natural support for the immune system, helping children stay healthy and resilient year-round.

Digestive Health: Gentle herbs like ginger, fennel, and chamomile can soothe upset stomachs, ease digestive discomfort, and promote healthy digestion in children. Whether it's calming colic in infants or easing indigestion in older children, these herbal remedies offer gentle relief for common digestive woes.

Sleep and Relaxation: Herbs like lavender, chamomile, and passionflower have long been valued for their calming and sedative effects, helping children relax and unwind before bedtime. These botanical allies can promote restful sleep and ease bedtime struggles, fostering a sense of peace and tranquility for both children and parents alike.

Empowering Parents with Herbal Wisdom

As we journey into the realm of herbs for children's health, we invite parents to embrace the gentle wisdom of nature and explore the healing wonders that botanical remedies have to offer. By integrating herbs into their children's daily routines, parents can nourish their little ones' bodies, minds, and spirits, fostering resilience, vitality, and well-being from the earliest stages of life. With each sip of herbal tea, each soothing bath, and each lovingly prepared remedy, parents can cultivate a deeper connection to the healing power of nature, empowering their children to thrive with vitality and joy, in harmony with the natural world.

Safe Herbal Remedies for Children: Nurturing Health with Nature's Gentle Touch

Introduction

In the delicate dance of childhood, where each step is a journey of discovery and wonder, parents seek to provide their little ones with the gentlest care possible. As advocates for their children's well-being, parents often turn to nature's pharmacy, seeking herbal remedies that offer comfort and relief without the harshness of synthetic chemicals. In this chapter, we explore a selection of safe and effective herbal remedies for children, empowering parents to nurture their children's health with the gentle touch of nature.

Understanding Safety in Herbal Remedies for Children

Dosage and Dilution: When administering herbal remedies to children, it is essential to consider their age, weight, and individual health needs. Herbal preparations should be appropriately dosed and diluted to ensure safety and efficacy, with careful attention paid to recommended dosages and administration methods.

Quality and Purity: The quality and purity of herbal remedies play a crucial role in their safety and effectiveness for children. Parents should source herbs from reputable suppliers who prioritize quality control and adhere to strict standards of purity and potency. Organic and wildcrafted herbs are often preferred to minimize the risk of exposure to pesticides and contaminants.

Consultation with Healthcare Providers: While many herbal remedies are safe for children when used appropriately, it is essential for parents to consult with qualified healthcare providers before administering herbal remedies, especially if their child has underlying health conditions or is taking medications. Healthcare providers can offer guidance on the safety, dosage, and suitability of herbal remedies for children based on individual health needs.

Safe Herbal Remedies for Common Childhood Ailments

Chamomile: Chamomile is prized for its gentle sedative and calming effects, making it a soothing remedy for children's sleep disturbances, teething discomfort, and digestive upset. Chamomile tea can be administered orally or used topically as a gentle wash for skin irritations and minor wounds.

Ginger: Ginger is renowned for its ability to soothe upset stomachs, relieve nausea, and alleviate motion sickness in children. Ginger tea or ginger-infused foods can be safely administered to children to ease digestive discomfort and promote healthy digestion.

Elderberry: Elderberry is a potent immune-boosting herb that can help strengthen children's defenses against colds, flu, and other respiratory infections. Elderberry syrup or elderberry-infused teas are safe and effective remedies for supporting children's immune health during cold and flu season.

Calendula: Calendula is a gentle and soothing herb with anti-inflammatory and antimicrobial properties, making it an ideal remedy for children's skin irritations, rashes, and minor cuts and scrapes. Calendula-infused creams, ointments, or salves can be applied topically to promote healing and relieve discomfort.

Nettle: Nettle is a nourishing herb rich in vitamins, minerals, and antioxidants, making it a valuable tonic for children's overall health and well-being. Nettle tea or nettle-infused foods can be safely incorporated into children's diets to support healthy growth and development.

As stewards of their children's health and well-being, parents have the privilege and responsibility to explore the gentle healing wonders of nature's herbal remedies. By selecting safe and effective herbal remedies and administering them with care and diligence, parents can nurture their children's health and vitality, fostering resilience, balance, and well-being from infancy through childhood. With each gentle remedy and loving touch, parents can cultivate a deeper connection to the healing power of nature, empowering their children to thrive with vitality and joy, in harmony with the natural world.

Treating Common Childhood Ailments with Gentle Herbal Remedies

Introduction

In the tender embrace of childhood, where laughter and exploration abound, little ones may occasionally encounter the discomforts and challenges of common ailments. As guardians of their well-being, parents seek gentle and effective remedies to alleviate their children's symptoms and restore their vibrant health. In this chapter, we explore a selection of herbal remedies that offer safe and soothing relief for common childhood ailments, empowering parents to nurture their children's health with the healing touch of nature.

Common Childhood Ailments and Herbal Solutions

Coughs and Colds: When cold and flu season arrives, children may experience coughs, congestion, and runny noses. Herbal remedies such as elderberry syrup, honey and lemon tea, and thyme-infused steam inhalations can help alleviate symptoms, soothe irritated throats, and support respiratory health.

Teething Discomfort: Teething can be a challenging time for both children and parents, with symptoms such as gum pain, irritability, and drooling. Herbal remedies such as chamomile tea, ginger-infused teething biscuits, and clove-infused oil can provide natural relief, soothing sore gums and calming fussiness.

Digestive Upset: Children may experience occasional digestive discomfort, including bloating, gas, and stomachaches, often due to dietary changes or mild illnesses. Herbal remedies such as ginger tea, fennel seed water, and chamomile-infused tummy rubs can help ease symptoms, promote healthy digestion, and soothe upset stomachs.

Skin Irritations: From minor cuts and scrapes to insect bites and rashes, children's skin can be prone to irritation and inflammation. Herbal remedies such as calendula salve, lavender-infused bathwater, and chamomile tea compresses can help soothe skin irritations, promote healing, and reduce discomfort.

Sleep Disturbances: Children may experience difficulty falling asleep or staying asleep due to stress, excitement, or disruptions to their bedtime routine. Herbal remedies such as lavender-infused pillows, chamomile tea, and passionflower tincture can help promote relaxation, calm the mind, and support restful sleep.

Guidelines for Herbal Remedies

Dosage and Administration: When administering herbal remedies to children, it is essential to follow recommended dosage guidelines and administration methods to ensure safety and effectiveness. Herbal teas can be diluted with water or juice, tinctures can be mixed into beverages, and topical remedies can be applied with gentle massage.

Quality and Safety: Choose high-quality, organic herbs from reputable sources to ensure purity and potency. Avoid herbs that may be toxic or unsuitable for children, and consult with a healthcare provider if you have any concerns about the safety or suitability of herbal remedies for your child.

Monitoring and Observation: Pay close attention to your child's response to herbal remedies, monitoring for any adverse reactions or changes in symptoms. Discontinue use and consult with a healthcare provider if you notice any unexpected or concerning effects.

With their gentle and nurturing qualities, herbal remedies offer safe and effective solutions for alleviating common childhood ailments and promoting overall well-being. By incorporating herbal remedies into their children's care routines, parents can provide gentle and holistic support for their children's health, fostering resilience, vitality, and joy from infancy through childhood. With each soothing sip of herbal tea, each comforting application of herbal salve, parents can cultivate a deeper connection to the healing power of nature, empowering their children to thrive with health and happiness, in harmony with the natural world.

Chamomile: Soothing Relief for Colic and Restful Sleep in Children

Introduction

In the tender moments of infancy, when the world is still new and every sensation is a discovery, babies may encounter the discomfort of colic and the challenge of settling into restful sleep. As caregivers, parents seek gentle and effective remedies to provide relief and promote tranquility for their little ones. In this chapter, we explore the calming virtues of chamomile, a cherished herb renowned for its ability to soothe colic and induce restful sleep in children, offering parents a comforting ally in their journey of nurturing their children's health and well-being.

Chamomile for Colic Relief

Understanding Colic: Colic is a common condition characterized by excessive crying, fussiness, and discomfort in infants, often occurring in the first few months of life. While the exact cause of colic remains unclear, factors such as digestive issues, gas, and overstimulation may contribute to its onset.

Soothing Properties of Chamomile: Chamomile is revered for its gentle and calming properties, making it a valuable remedy for soothing colicky babies. The herb's anti-inflammatory and antispasmodic effects help relax the digestive tract, ease gas and bloating, and reduce discomfort associated with colic.

Administration of Chamomile for Colic: Chamomile can be administered to colicky babies in various forms, including chamomile tea, chamomile-infused gripe water, and chamomile tummy rubs. A few drops of chamomile tea or diluted chamomile tincture can be given orally to infants, while chamomile-infused gripe water can be administered with a dropper before or after feedings to alleviate digestive discomfort.

Chamomile for Restful Sleep

Promoting Sleep in Children: Sleep is essential for the growth, development, and well-being of children, yet many babies and young children struggle to settle into restful sleep. Chamomile offers a gentle and natural solution for promoting relaxation, calming the mind, and inducing restful sleep in children.

Soothing Bedtime Rituals: Incorporating chamomile into bedtime rituals can help signal to children that it is time to unwind and prepare for sleep. A warm chamomile bath, chamomile-infused massage oil, or a cup of chamomile tea can all serve as soothing rituals to promote relaxation and tranquility before bedtime.

Calming Effects of Chamomile: Chamomile contains compounds such as apigenin and bisabolol, which exert sedative and anxiolytic effects, helping to reduce anxiety, promote relaxation, and facilitate the onset of sleep. The herb's gentle and mild flavor makes it a palatable and well-tolerated remedy for children of all ages.

Guidelines for Safe Use

Dosage and Dilution: When administering chamomile to infants and young children, it is essential to dilute the herb appropriately and follow recommended dosage guidelines to ensure safety and effectiveness. Chamomile tea can be diluted with breast milk, formula, or water, while chamomile tinctures should be diluted according to the manufacturer's instructions.

Quality and Purity: Choose high-quality, organic chamomile from reputable sources to ensure purity and potency. Avoid chamomile products that contain additives, preservatives, or artificial flavors, and opt for whole chamomile flowers or loose-leaf chamomile tea for optimal freshness and efficacy.

Consultation with Healthcare Providers: While chamomile is generally considered safe for most infants and children, it is always advisable to consult with a healthcare provider before using herbal remedies, especially in cases of underlying health conditions or allergies. Healthcare providers can offer guidance on the safety, dosage, and suitability of chamomile for individual children based on their unique health needs.

Chamomile, with its gentle and soothing properties, offers parents a natural and effective remedy for soothing colic and promoting restful sleep in children. By incorporating chamomile into their care routines, parents can provide comfort, relief, and tranquility for their little ones, fostering health, well-being, and harmony in the early stages of life. With each sip of chamomile tea, each lovingly administered tummy rub, parents can cultivate a deeper connection to the healing power of nature, empowering their children to thrive with peace and vitality, in harmony with the natural world.

Fennel: Nature's Remedy for Digestive Comfort

Introduction

In the delicate balance of childhood, digestive discomfort can disrupt the tranquility of daily life, causing discomfort and distress for little ones and concern for their caregivers. Seeking gentle and effective solutions, parents turn to the soothing properties of fennel, a cherished herb renowned for its ability to calm upset stomachs and ease digestive issues in children. In this chapter, we explore the digestive virtues of fennel, offering parents a natural and comforting ally in nurturing their children's digestive health and well-being.

Understanding Digestive Issues in Children

Common Digestive Complaints: Children may experience a range of digestive issues, including gas, bloating, indigestion, and stomachaches, often resulting from dietary indiscretions, food intolerances, or mild illnesses. These digestive discomforts can cause distress and disrupt children's daily activities, affecting their overall well-being and quality of life.

Importance of Digestive Health: Optimal digestive health is essential for children's growth, development, and well-being, as it allows for the proper absorption of nutrients, supports immune function, and contributes to overall vitality and vitality. Addressing digestive issues promptly and effectively can help children feel more comfortable, energetic, and resilient in their daily lives.

Fennel: A Gentle Remedy for Digestive Comfort

Soothing Properties of Fennel: Fennel (Foeniculum vulgare) is esteemed for its gentle and carminative properties, making it a valuable remedy for soothing digestive discomfort and promoting gastrointestinal health in children. The herb's volatile oils, including anethole, fenchone, and estragole, help relax the smooth muscles of the digestive tract, reduce gas formation, and ease bloating and cramping.

Alleviating Digestive Discomfort: Fennel is commonly used to alleviate a variety of digestive issues in children, including colic, gas, bloating, indigestion, and stomachaches. The herb's soothing and anti-inflammatory effects help calm irritated stomachs, promote healthy digestion, and alleviate discomfort associated with common digestive complaints.

Administering Fennel for Digestive Relief

Fennel Tea: Fennel tea is a simple and effective remedy for soothing digestive discomfort in children. To prepare fennel tea, steep crushed fennel seeds in hot water for 5-10 minutes, then strain and allow the tea to cool to a safe temperature before offering it to your child to drink. Fennel tea can be sweetened with a touch of honey for added palatability.

Fennel Water: Fennel water is a gentle and hydrating remedy that can be given to infants and young children to alleviate digestive discomfort. To make fennel water, steep crushed fennel seeds in boiled water, then allow the mixture to cool before offering it to your child in small, frequent doses throughout the day.

Fennel Infused Foods: Fennel can be incorporated into your child's diet in various ways to promote digestive health and alleviate discomfort. Fennel seeds can be added to soups, stews, and cooked grains, while fennel bulb can be roasted, sautéed, or pureed into soups and sauces for added flavor and nutrition.

Guidelines for Safe Use

Dosage and Dilution: When administering fennel to children, it is essential to use an appropriate dosage and dilution to ensure safety and effectiveness. Fennel tea can be diluted with water or milk for infants and young children, while older children may consume stronger preparations as needed.

Quality and Purity: Choose high-quality, organic fennel seeds from reputable sources to ensure purity and potency. Avoid fennel products that contain additives, preservatives, or artificial flavors, and opt for whole fennel seeds or freshly ground fennel powder for optimal freshness and efficacy.

Consultation with Healthcare Providers: While fennel is generally considered safe for most children, it is advisable to consult with a healthcare provider before using herbal remedies, especially in cases of underlying health conditions or allergies. Healthcare providers can offer guidance on the safety, dosage, and suitability of fennel for individual children based on their unique health needs.

Fennel, with its gentle and carminative properties, offers parents a natural and effective remedy for soothing digestive discomfort and promoting gastrointestinal health in children. By incorporating fennel into their care routines, parents can provide comfort, relief, and digestive support for their little ones, fostering health, well-being, and vitality in the early stages of life. With each sip of fennel tea, each lovingly prepared meal infused with fennel flavor, parents can cultivate a deeper connection to the healing power of nature, empowering their children to thrive with comfort and resilience, in harmony with the natural world.

Licorice Root: Soothing Relief for Coughs

Introduction

In the symphony of childhood, where laughter and play abound, the occasional cough may disrupt the harmony, causing discomfort and concern for both children and their caregivers. Seeking gentle and effective remedies, parents turn to the soothing properties of licorice root, a cherished herb revered for its ability to calm coughs and ease respiratory distress. In this chapter, we explore the cough-relieving virtues of licorice root, offering parents a natural and comforting ally in nurturing their children's respiratory health and well-being.

Understanding Coughs in Children

Common Respiratory Ailment: Coughing is a common symptom of respiratory infections, allergies, and irritants, often causing discomfort and distress for children. While coughing serves as a protective mechanism to clear the airways of mucus and foreign particles, persistent or severe coughs can interfere with sleep, eating, and daily activities.

Types of Coughs: Coughs can be characterized as dry or productive (wet), depending on the presence of mucus. Dry coughs are often caused by irritation or inflammation of the throat and airways, while productive coughs help expel mucus and debris from the respiratory tract.

Licorice Root: Nature's Soother for Cough Relief

Demulcent and Expectorant Properties: Licorice root (Glycyrrhiza glabra) is esteemed for its demulcent and expectorant properties, making it an invaluable remedy for soothing dry coughs and promoting expectoration in children. The herb's mucilaginous compounds help coat and soothe the throat and airways, while its expectorant action helps loosen and expel mucus from the respiratory tract.

Anti-inflammatory Effects: Licorice root contains anti-inflammatory compounds, including glycyrrhizin, which help reduce inflammation and irritation in the respiratory tract. By calming inflamed tissues and reducing cough reflex sensitivity, licorice root provides relief from cough-related discomfort and promotes respiratory comfort.

Administering Licorice Root for Cough Relief

Licorice Tea: Licorice tea is a simple and effective remedy for soothing dry coughs and promoting respiratory comfort in children. To prepare licorice tea, steep licorice root slices or dried licorice root in hot water for 5-10 minutes, then strain and allow the tea to cool to a safe temperature before offering it to your child to drink.

Licorice Syrup: Licorice syrup combines the soothing properties of licorice root with the sweetness of honey or other natural sweeteners, making it a palatable and kid-friendly remedy for cough relief. Licorice syrup can be administered orally to children in small, frequent doses throughout the day to soothe dry coughs and promote respiratory comfort.

Licorice Lozenges: Licorice lozenges provide a convenient and portable option for cough relief on the go. Made with licorice root extract and natural sweeteners, licorice lozenges help soothe throat irritation, suppress cough reflex sensitivity, and promote respiratory comfort in children.

Guidelines for Safe Use

Dosage and Frequency: When administering licorice root to children, it is essential to use an appropriate dosage and frequency to ensure safety and effectiveness. Licorice tea and syrup can be given to children in small, frequent doses throughout the day as needed to alleviate cough-related discomfort.

Quality and Purity: Choose high-quality, organic licorice root products from reputable sources to ensure purity and potency. Avoid licorice products that contain additives, preservatives, or artificial flavors, and opt for whole licorice root or licorice root extracts derived from reputable suppliers for optimal efficacy.

Consultation with Healthcare Providers: While licorice root is generally considered safe for most children, it is advisable to consult with a healthcare provider before using herbal remedies, especially in cases of underlying health conditions or allergies. Healthcare providers can offer guidance on the safety, dosage, and suitability of licorice root for individual children based on their unique health needs.

Licorice root, with its soothing and expectorant properties, offers parents a natural and effective remedy for relieving coughs and promoting respiratory comfort in children. By incorporating licorice root into their care routines, parents can provide gentle and nurturing support for their children's respiratory health, helping them breathe easier and feel more comfortable. With each sip of licorice tea, each spoonful of licorice syrup, parents can cultivate a deeper connection to the healing power of nature, empowering their children to thrive with vitality and well-being, in harmony with the natural world.

Exploring Special Topics in Herbal Medicine: Navigating the Depths of Natural Healing

Introduction

As we journey deeper into the realm of herbal medicine, we encounter a diverse array of topics that offer insight, inspiration, and innovation in the pursuit of holistic health and well-being. In this chapter, we embark on a voyage of exploration, delving into special topics in herbal medicine that illuminate the multifaceted nature of natural healing. From ancient traditions to modern applications, from common ailments to specialized conditions, we uncover the richness and depth of herbal medicine's vast terrain, inviting readers to discover new perspectives, deepen their understanding, and expand their toolkit for optimal health and vitality.

The Tapestry of Herbal Medicine

Ancient Wisdom: Herbal medicine traces its roots back to ancient civilizations, where healers and herbalists relied on the healing properties of plants to promote health and treat illness. Drawing upon centuries of accumulated knowledge and wisdom, traditional herbal medicine offers a treasure trove of remedies and practices that continue to inspire and inform modern herbalists and healthcare practitioners.

Modern Science: In the age of scientific inquiry, herbal medicine undergoes rigorous scrutiny and investigation, with researchers exploring the pharmacological properties, mechanisms of action, and clinical efficacy of medicinal plants. Through laboratory studies, clinical trials, and evidence-based research, modern science sheds light on the therapeutic potential of herbal remedies, validating their use and expanding their applications in contemporary healthcare.

Exploring Special Topics

Herbs for Women's Health: From menstrual cramps to menopausal symptoms, herbs play a vital role in supporting women's health and well-being throughout all stages of life. We delve into the unique properties of herbs such as chasteberry, dong quai, and red raspberry leaf, exploring their therapeutic effects on hormonal balance, reproductive health, and menstrual cycle regulation.

Herbal Solutions for Children's Health: Children's health presents its own set of challenges and considerations, calling for gentle yet effective remedies that support growth, development, and vitality. We uncover the soothing properties of herbs like chamomile, fennel, and licorice root, offering safe and natural solutions for common childhood ailments such as colic, coughs, and digestive discomfort.

Herbal Remedies for Chronic Conditions: Chronic conditions such as arthritis, diabetes, and cardiovascular disease require comprehensive management strategies that address underlying imbalances and promote long-term wellness. We explore the role of herbs such as turmeric, fenugreek, and hawthorn in managing chronic conditions, highlighting their anti-inflammatory, blood sugar-regulating, and cardiovascular-supporting properties.

Herbal Allies for Mental Health: In the realm of mental health and emotional well-being, herbs offer gentle yet powerful support for managing stress, anxiety, and depression. We delve into the calming effects of herbs like ashwagandha, valerian, and lemon balm, exploring their adaptogenic, anxiolytic, and mood-stabilizing properties that help promote inner peace and emotional resilience.

As we navigate the special topics in herbal medicine, we uncover a tapestry of traditions, innovations, and insights that illuminate the path to optimal health and vitality. Whether exploring ancient wisdom or embracing modern science, whether addressing common ailments or specialized conditions, herbal medicine offers a holistic approach to healing that honors the interconnectedness of body, mind, and spirit. With each exploration and discovery, readers are invited to deepen their appreciation for the healing power of nature and embrace the transformative potential of herbal medicine in their journey toward wellness and wholeness.

Harnessing Nature's Cleansing Power: Herbs for Detoxification

Introduction

In our modern world filled with environmental pollutants, processed foods, and daily stressors, the body's natural detoxification systems can become overwhelmed, leading to a buildup of toxins and impurities that compromise health and vitality. Fortunately, the healing power of nature offers a multitude of herbs that support the body's detoxification processes, helping to cleanse, rejuvenate, and restore balance from within. In this chapter, we explore the transformative properties of herbs for detoxification, offering a holistic approach to purifying the body, refreshing the mind, and revitalizing the spirit.

Understanding Detoxification

The Body's Innate Wisdom: The human body possesses remarkable self-cleansing mechanisms, including the liver, kidneys, lungs, skin, and lymphatic system, which work synergistically to eliminate toxins and waste products from the body. However, in today's toxic environment, these systems can become overwhelmed, leading to a buildup of toxins that impair cellular function and compromise overall health.

The Importance of Detoxification: Detoxification is essential for maintaining health and vitality, as it allows the body to eliminate harmful substances, neutralize free radicals, and support optimal organ function. By supporting the body's natural detoxification pathways, individuals can experience increased energy, improved digestion, clearer skin, and enhanced overall well-being.

Herbs for Detoxification

Dandelion: Dandelion (Taraxacum officinale) is revered for its potent detoxifying properties, particularly its ability to support liver health and bile production. Rich in antioxidants and bitter compounds, dandelion helps stimulate liver function, enhance bile flow, and promote the elimination of toxins from the body.

Milk Thistle: Milk thistle (Silybum marianum) is renowned for its protective effects on the liver, making it a valuable herb for detoxification. The active compound in milk thistle, silymarin, helps regenerate liver cells, reduce inflammation, and enhance detoxification pathways, thereby supporting overall liver health and function.

Burdock Root: Burdock root (Arctium lappa) is prized for its blood-purifying properties, making it an excellent herb for detoxification. Rich in antioxidants and anti-inflammatory compounds, burdock root helps cleanse the blood, promote lymphatic drainage, and support the elimination of toxins through the skin, kidneys, and liver.

Nettle: Nettle (Urtica dioica) is a nourishing herb rich in vitamins, minerals, and phytonutrients that support detoxification and overall health. Nettle helps cleanse the blood, support kidney function, and promote the elimination of waste products, making it an ideal herb for supporting the body's natural detoxification processes.

Incorporating Herbs into Your Detoxification Routine

Herbal Teas: Enjoying herbal teas made from dandelion, milk thistle, burdock root, and nettle is a simple and effective way to incorporate detoxifying herbs into your daily routine. These teas can be enjoyed hot or cold and can be sweetened with honey or lemon for added flavor.

Herbal Tinctures: Herbal tinctures made from detoxifying herbs can be taken orally to support liver function, promote lymphatic drainage, and enhance the body's natural detoxification processes. Tinctures can be diluted in water or juice and taken daily as part of a comprehensive detoxification regimen.

Herbal Supplements: Herbal supplements containing detoxifying herbs such as dandelion, milk thistle, burdock root, and nettle are available in various forms, including capsules, tablets, and powders. These supplements can be taken daily to support detoxification and overall health, particularly during times of increased toxin exposure or stress.

Guidelines for Safe Detoxification

Hydration: Stay well-hydrated by drinking plenty of water throughout the day to support the body's natural detoxification processes and facilitate the elimination of toxins.

Nutrient-Rich Diet: Eat a balanced diet rich in fruits, vegetables, whole grains, and lean proteins to provide essential nutrients that support detoxification and overall health.

Gentle Exercise: Engage in regular physical activity, such as walking, yoga, or swimming, to promote circulation, lymphatic drainage, and the elimination of toxins through sweat and respiration.

Consultation with Healthcare Providers: Before embarking on a detoxification regimen, especially if you have underlying health conditions or are taking medications, consult with a healthcare provider to ensure that detoxification is safe and appropriate for your individual needs.

Herbs for detoxification offer a gentle yet potent approach to cleansing the body, refreshing the mind, and revitalizing the spirit. By incorporating detoxifying herbs into your daily routine and supporting the body's natural cleansing processes, you can experience increased energy, improved digestion, clearer skin, and enhanced overall well-being. With each sip of herbal tea, each dose of herbal tincture, you embark on a journey of renewal and transformation, embracing the healing power of nature and nurturing your body, mind, and spirit back to balance and vitality.

Dandelion: Nature's Liver Tonic

Dandelion (Taraxacum officinale)

Introduction

Often dismissed as a pesky weed, the dandelion plant, with its cheerful yellow flowers and jagged leaves, is a powerhouse of nutrition and healing. Revered for centuries in traditional medicine systems worldwide, dandelion offers a plethora of health benefits, particularly for liver health and detoxification. In this exploration, we uncover the remarkable properties of dandelion and its role as nature's liver tonic.

Nutritional Profile

Dandelion is packed with essential nutrients, including vitamins A, C, and K, as well as minerals like iron, calcium, and potassium. Its leaves are rich in antioxidants and bitter compounds, while its roots contain inulin, a prebiotic fiber that supports gut health.

Liver Support

Dandelion leaves: The bitter compounds in dandelion leaves stimulate bile production and flow, aiding digestion and promoting liver function. By supporting the liver's detoxification pathways, dandelion leaves help eliminate toxins and waste products from the body, promoting overall well-being.

Dandelion roots: Dandelion roots contain compounds called sesquiterpene lactones, which have been shown to protect the liver from oxidative stress and inflammation. Additionally, dandelion roots support liver regeneration and may help alleviate symptoms of liver congestion and sluggishness.

Detoxification

Dandelion's diuretic properties promote the elimination of excess fluids and toxins from the body through urine. This helps reduce bloating, water retention, and swelling, while also supporting kidney function and urinary tract health.

Supporting Digestion

Dandelion's bitter compounds stimulate digestive juices, including saliva, stomach acid, and bile, enhancing digestion and nutrient absorption. This can help alleviate symptoms of indigestion, bloating, and constipation, promoting overall digestive health.

Incorporating Dandelion into Your Routine

Dandelion tea: Steep dandelion leaves or roots in hot water to make a nourishing and detoxifying herbal tea. Enjoy it alone or blend it with other herbs for added flavor and benefits.

Dandelion salad: Add fresh dandelion leaves to salads for a nutritious and flavorful boost. Pair them with other greens, vegetables, and a tangy dressing for a refreshing and revitalizing meal.

Dandelion supplements: Dandelion supplements, including capsules, tablets, and tinctures, are available for those who prefer a more concentrated form of dandelion's therapeutic benefits. Follow dosage recommendations and consult with a healthcare provider if needed.

Safety Considerations

While generally safe for most people, dandelion may cause allergic reactions in individuals sensitive to plants in the Asteraceae family. Pregnant or breastfeeding women should consult with a healthcare provider before using dandelion supplements. Additionally, individuals with gallbladder issues or bile duct obstruction should avoid dandelion due to its bile-stimulating effects.

Dandelion, often overlooked and underappreciated, emerges as a potent ally for liver health, detoxification, and digestion. By incorporating dandelion into your daily routine, whether through teas, salads, or supplements, you can harness its remarkable healing properties and support your body's natural detoxification processes. With each sip of dandelion tea, each bite of dandelion salad, you nourish your body, revitalize your liver, and embrace the abundant gifts of nature's humble weed.

Milk Thistle: Guardian of Liver Health

Milk Thistle (Silybum marianum)

Introduction

Nestled within the vibrant world of herbal remedies, milk thistle stands tall as a stalwart guardian of liver health. With its striking purple flowers and glossy green leaves, this herb has been revered for centuries for its remarkable ability to support liver function and protect against liver damage. In this exploration, we uncover the secrets of milk thistle and its role as nature's liver protector.

Nutritional Profile

Milk thistle seeds contain a powerhouse of bioactive compounds, most notably silymarin, a flavonoid complex with potent antioxidant and anti-inflammatory properties. Silymarin is the key to milk thistle's liver-protective effects, offering support and rejuvenation to this vital organ.

Liver Support

Silymarin: The active compound in milk thistle, silymarin, acts as a potent antioxidant, scavenging free radicals and reducing oxidative stress in the liver. By protecting liver cells from damage and promoting their regeneration, silymarin helps maintain optimal liver function and vitality.

Detoxification: Milk thistle supports the liver's natural detoxification processes, enhancing the elimination of toxins, pollutants, and metabolic waste products from the body. This helps lighten the liver's burden and promotes overall well-being.

Liver Conditions

Liver Diseases: Milk thistle is particularly beneficial for individuals with liver conditions such as fatty liver disease, hepatitis, and cirrhosis. Studies have shown that milk thistle may help reduce inflammation, improve liver function tests, and slow the progression of liver disease in some cases.

Liver Protection: In addition to supporting liver health in individuals with existing liver conditions, milk thistle may also offer protection against liver damage from environmental toxins, alcohol, medications, and other factors. Its antioxidant and anti-inflammatory properties help shield liver cells from harm and maintain their integrity.

Digestive Support

Mild Laxative: Milk thistle has a mild laxative effect, promoting bowel regularity and easing digestive discomfort. By supporting healthy digestion and elimination, milk thistle contributes to overall digestive well-being.

Incorporating Milk Thistle into Your Routine

Milk Thistle Supplements: Milk thistle supplements, available in capsules, tablets, and tinctures, provide a convenient way to incorporate this herb into your daily routine. Follow dosage recommendations and consult with a healthcare provider if needed.

Milk Thistle Tea: Steep milk thistle seeds or leaves in hot water to make a nourishing and liver-protective herbal tea. Enjoy it alone or blend it with other herbs for added flavor and benefits.

Safety Considerations

Milk thistle is generally considered safe for most people when taken in recommended doses. However, individuals with allergies to plants in the Asteraceae family should avoid milk thistle. Pregnant or breastfeeding women should consult with a healthcare provider before using milk thistle supplements.

Milk thistle stands as a stalwart guardian of liver health, offering protection, support, and rejuvenation to this vital organ. By incorporating milk thistle into your daily routine, whether through supplements or teas, you can harness its remarkable healing properties and promote optimal liver function and vitality. With each dose of milk thistle, you nourish your liver, protect your health, and embrace the abundance of nature's healing gifts.

Burdock Root: Nature's Blood Purifier and Skin Healer

Burdock Root (Arctium lappa)

Introduction

In the realm of herbal medicine, burdock root stands out as a humble yet powerful ally for cleansing the blood, supporting digestion, and promoting radiant skin. With its long taproot and broad leaves, this unassuming plant holds a wealth of therapeutic properties that have been revered for centuries in traditional healing practices. In this exploration, we uncover the secrets of burdock root and its role as nature's blood purifier and skin healer.

Nutritional Profile

Burdock root is rich in essential nutrients, including vitamins B6 and C, potassium, iron, and manganese. It also contains a unique combination of bioactive compounds, including lignans, inulin, and polyphenols, which contribute to its medicinal properties.

Blood Purification

Burdock root: The bitter compounds in burdock root stimulate digestion and promote the elimination of toxins from the body. As a blood purifier, burdock root helps remove metabolic waste products, environmental toxins, and excess hormones from the bloodstream, supporting overall health and vitality.

Lymphatic Support: Burdock root supports lymphatic drainage, helping to remove toxins and waste products from the lymphatic system. By promoting lymphatic circulation, burdock root reduces congestion and swelling in the lymph nodes, supporting immune function and detoxification.

Skin Health

Burdock root: The anti-inflammatory and antibacterial properties of burdock root make it an excellent remedy for various skin conditions, including acne, eczema, psoriasis, and dermatitis. By reducing inflammation, soothing irritation, and inhibiting bacterial growth, burdock root helps promote clear, healthy skin.

Antioxidant Protection: Burdock root is rich in antioxidants, which help neutralize free radicals and protect skin cells from oxidative damage. This helps prevent premature aging, wrinkles, and other signs of skin aging, promoting a youthful and radiant complexion.

Digestive Support

Burdock root: The bitter compounds in burdock root stimulate digestive juices, including saliva, stomach acid, and bile, enhancing digestion and nutrient absorption. This can help alleviate symptoms of indigestion, bloating, and constipation, promoting overall digestive health.

Incorporating Burdock Root into Your Routine

Burdock root tea: Steep dried burdock root slices or powder in hot water to make a nourishing and detoxifying herbal tea. Enjoy it alone or blend it with other herbs for added flavor and benefits.

Burdock root supplements: Burdock root supplements, available in capsules, tablets, and tinctures, provide a convenient way to incorporate this herb into your daily routine. Follow dosage recommendations and consult with a healthcare provider if needed.

Safety Considerations

Burdock root is generally considered safe for most people when taken in recommended doses. However, individuals with allergies to plants in the Asteraceae family should avoid burdock root. Pregnant or breastfeeding women should consult with a healthcare provider before using burdock root supplements.

Burdock root emerges as a versatile and potent ally for blood purification, skin health, and digestive support. By incorporating burdock root into your daily routine, whether through teas or supplements, you can harness its remarkable healing properties and promote overall health and vitality. With each sip of burdock root tea, each dose of burdock root supplement, you nourish your body, cleanse your blood, and embrace the abundant gifts of nature's healing bounty.

Cilantro: A Culinary Herb with Remarkable Health Benefits

Cilantro (Coriandrum sativum)

Introduction

Cilantro, also known as coriander in some regions, is a beloved culinary herb prized for its fresh and citrusy flavor. Beyond its culinary uses, cilantro boasts a wealth of health benefits, ranging from detoxification and digestion support to anti-inflammatory and antimicrobial properties. In this exploration, we uncover the secrets of cilantro and its role as a versatile herb for both culinary delight and therapeutic wellness.

Nutritional Profile

Cilantro is rich in vitamins, minerals, and phytonutrients that contribute to its health-promoting properties. It is particularly high in vitamins A and K, as well as antioxidants such as beta-carotene and lutein. Additionally, cilantro contains essential minerals like potassium, calcium, and magnesium.

Detoxification

Cilantro: The unique compounds in cilantro, including chlorophyll and certain volatile oils, have been shown to bind to heavy metals and other toxins in the body, aiding in their removal through urine and feces. This makes cilantro an excellent herb for detoxification and cleansing.

Digestive Support

Cilantro: The essential oils in cilantro, such as linalool and geranyl acetate, have been found to promote healthy digestion by stimulating digestive enzymes and reducing gas and bloating. Additionally, cilantro's antimicrobial properties help combat harmful bacteria in the digestive tract, supporting gut health.

Anti-Inflammatory Effects

Cilantro: Certain compounds in cilantro, such as quercetin and kaempferol, possess anti-inflammatory properties that may help reduce inflammation in the body. This can be beneficial for conditions such as arthritis, allergies, and inflammatory bowel diseases.

Antimicrobial Properties

Cilantro: Cilantro contains natural antimicrobial compounds, including dodecenal and cineole, which have been shown to inhibit the growth of bacteria and fungi. This makes cilantro a valuable herb for preserving food and supporting oral health.

Incorporating Cilantro into Your Diet

Culinary Uses: Cilantro adds a burst of fresh flavor to a wide variety of dishes, including salads, salsas, soups, curries, and marinades. It pairs well with ingredients like lime, garlic, ginger, and chili peppers, enhancing the taste and aroma of dishes.

Cilantro Pesto: Blend fresh cilantro leaves with garlic, olive oil, nuts (such as almonds or pine nuts), and Parmesan cheese to make a delicious and nutritious cilantro pesto. Use it as a sauce for pasta, spread for sandwiches, or dip for vegetables.

Safety Considerations

While cilantro is generally safe for most people when consumed in culinary amounts, some individuals may experience allergic reactions or digestive upset. It is also important to source cilantro from reputable sources to avoid potential contamination with pesticides or heavy metals.

Cilantro, with its vibrant flavor and impressive health benefits, is a true gem in the world of culinary herbs. By incorporating cilantro into your diet on a regular basis, whether as a garnish, seasoning, or main ingredient, you can enjoy its delicious taste while reaping the rewards of its therapeutic properties. With each bite of cilantro-laced cuisine, you nourish your body, delight your taste buds, and embrace the abundance of nature's culinary and medicinal bounty.

Enhancing Physical Performance with Herbs and Supplements

Introduction

In the pursuit of peak physical performance, athletes and fitness enthusiasts are constantly seeking ways to optimize their training, recovery, and overall health. While proper nutrition, training, and rest are essential components of performance enhancement, certain herbs and supplements have also gained popularity for their potential to support endurance, strength, and recovery. In this exploration, we delve into the realm of herbal remedies and supplements for enhancing physical performance, offering insights into their mechanisms of action and evidence-based benefits.

Herbs and Supplements for Performance Enhancement

1. Rhodiola Rosea: Rhodiola rosea, also known as golden root, is an adaptogenic herb revered for its ability to enhance endurance, reduce fatigue, and improve cognitive function. Studies suggest that rhodiola rosea may help increase oxygen utilization, regulate stress hormones, and enhance physical and mental performance during exercise.

2. Cordyceps: Cordyceps is a medicinal mushroom with adaptogenic and energizing properties. It has been traditionally used to improve stamina, endurance, and oxygen utilization, making it a popular choice among athletes and endurance enthusiasts. Cordyceps supplements are believed to enhance aerobic capacity, delay fatigue, and support overall physical performance.

3. Beetroot: Beetroot juice, rich in nitrates, has gained attention for its potential to enhance athletic performance. Nitrate-rich beetroot juice may help improve blood flow, reduce oxygen cost during exercise, and enhance exercise tolerance and performance, particularly during endurance activities such as running and cycling.

4. Creatine: Creatine is a naturally occurring compound found in muscle cells, where it plays a key role in energy production during short bursts of high-intensity exercise. Supplementing with creatine has been shown to increase muscle creatine stores, improve strength and power output, and enhance performance in activities requiring short bursts of maximal effort, such as weightlifting and sprinting.

5. Branched-Chain Amino Acids (BCAAs): BCAAs, including leucine, isoleucine, and valine, are essential amino acids that play crucial roles in muscle protein synthesis, energy production, and

recovery. Supplementing with BCAAs before or during exercise may help reduce muscle breakdown, delay fatigue, and promote recovery, particularly during prolonged or high-intensity workouts.

6. Beta-Alanine: Beta-alanine is a non-essential amino acid that combines with histidine to form carnosine, a dipeptide found in muscle tissue. Supplementation with beta-alanine has been shown to increase muscle carnosine levels, buffer lactic acid accumulation, and delay fatigue during high-intensity exercise, leading to improved performance in activities such as sprinting and interval training.

Incorporating Herbs and Supplements into Your Routine

Before incorporating herbs and supplements into your regimen, it is essential to consult with a healthcare professional or sports nutritionist to ensure safety and efficacy, particularly if you have underlying health conditions or are taking medications. Additionally, quality, purity, and dosage are crucial considerations when selecting herbal remedies and supplements, so be sure to choose reputable brands and follow recommended dosing guidelines.

Herbs and supplements offer promising avenues for enhancing physical performance, supporting endurance, strength, and recovery in athletes and fitness enthusiasts. By incorporating evidence-based remedies such as rhodiola rosea, cordyceps, beetroot, creatine, BCAAs, and beta-alanine into your training regimen, you can optimize your athletic performance and achieve your fitness goals with confidence and vitality. With each step, each lift, each breath, you harness the power of nature's bounty, unlocking your full potential and reaching new heights of physical excellence.

Ginseng: Nature's Energizing Elixir

Ginseng (Panax spp.)

Introduction

Ginseng, renowned for centuries in traditional Chinese medicine and beyond, stands as a symbol of vitality, resilience, and longevity. With its fleshy roots and distinctive aroma, ginseng has earned a reputation as a potent adaptogen, supporting overall health and well-being. In this exploration, we uncover the secrets of ginseng and its role as nature's energizing elixir.

Varieties of Ginseng

Panax ginseng (Asian or Korean ginseng): This variety of ginseng is native to East Asia and is the most widely researched and used species. It is revered for its energizing and revitalizing properties, supporting physical stamina, mental clarity, and overall vitality.

Panax quinquefolius (American ginseng): Indigenous to North America, American ginseng is prized for its calming and balancing effects. It is often used to support stress management, cognitive function, and immune health.

Siberian ginseng (Eleutherococcus senticosus): Despite its name, Siberian ginseng is not a true ginseng but shares similar adaptogenic properties. It is known for its ability to enhance resilience to stress, improve endurance, and support immune function.

Health Benefits of Ginseng

Adaptogenic Properties: Ginseng is classified as an adaptogen, a unique class of herbs that help the body adapt to stressors and restore balance. By modulating the body's stress response, ginseng supports resilience, vitality, and overall well-being.

Energy and Stamina: Ginseng is prized for its ability to enhance physical stamina, endurance, and performance. It helps increase energy levels, reduce fatigue, and improve exercise capacity, making it a popular choice among athletes and fitness enthusiasts.

Cognitive Function: Ginseng has been shown to support cognitive function, memory, and concentration. It may help enhance mental clarity, focus, and alertness, particularly during periods of stress or fatigue.

Immune Support: Ginseng contains compounds, such as ginsenosides, polysaccharides, and polyphenols, that support immune function and enhance resistance to infections. It helps strengthen the body's natural defenses, promoting overall immune health.

Stress Management: Ginseng's adaptogenic properties help mitigate the effects of stress on the body and mind. It helps reduce stress hormone levels, promote relaxation, and improve resilience to stressors, supporting mental and emotional well-being.

Incorporating Ginseng into Your Routine

Supplements: Ginseng supplements are available in various forms, including capsules, tablets, extracts, and powders. Choose high-quality products from reputable brands and follow recommended dosage guidelines.

Tea: Ginseng tea can be made by steeping dried ginseng root or ginseng tea bags in hot water. Enjoy it alone or blend it with other herbs for added flavor and benefits.

Tinctures: Ginseng tinctures are concentrated liquid extracts that can be added to water or juice for easy consumption. Follow dosage recommendations and consult with a healthcare professional if needed.

Safety Considerations

While ginseng is generally safe for most people when taken in recommended doses, it may interact with certain medications and health conditions. Consult with a healthcare professional before using ginseng supplements, especially if you have underlying health concerns or are taking prescription medications.

Ginseng, with its rich history and myriad health benefits, continues to captivate and inspire individuals seeking vitality, resilience, and well-being. By incorporating ginseng into your daily routine, whether through supplements, teas, or tinctures, you can harness its energizing and rejuvenating properties, supporting your body, mind, and spirit on the journey to optimal health and vitality. With each sip, each dose, you embrace the power of nature's timeless tonic, unlocking your full potential and embracing life with vigor and vitality.

Maca: Nature's Energizing Superfood

Maca (Lepidium meyenii)

Introduction

Nestled high in the Andes mountains of Peru, maca root has been treasured for centuries by indigenous cultures for its remarkable health-promoting properties. Revered as a sacred plant and a potent superfood, maca has earned a reputation as nature's energizing elixir, supporting vitality, stamina, and hormonal balance. In this exploration, we uncover the secrets of maca and its role as a powerhouse of nutrition and vitality.

Nutritional Profile

Maca root is rich in essential nutrients, including vitamins, minerals, and bioactive compounds that contribute to its health-promoting properties. It is particularly high in vitamin C, iron, potassium, and copper, as well as protein, fiber, and beneficial plant compounds like glucosinolates and polyphenols.

Health Benefits of Maca

Energy and Stamina: Maca is prized for its ability to increase energy levels, enhance endurance, and improve physical performance. It helps combat fatigue, reduce exercise-induced stress, and promote overall vitality, making it a popular choice among athletes and active individuals.

Hormonal Balance: Maca contains unique compounds known as macaenes and macamides, which have been shown to support hormonal balance and reproductive health. It may help regulate menstrual cycles, alleviate symptoms of menopause, and improve fertility in both men and women.

Stress Management: Maca is classified as an adaptogen, a special class of herbs that help the body adapt to stress and restore balance. It helps reduce stress hormone levels, promote relaxation, and improve resilience to physical and emotional stressors.

Libido and Sexual Health: Maca has a long history of use as an aphrodisiac and libido-enhancing herb. It may help improve sexual function, increase libido, and enhance sexual satisfaction in both men and women, making it a natural and safe alternative to conventional treatments for sexual dysfunction.

Cognitive Function: Maca's adaptogenic properties extend to cognitive function, memory, and mental clarity. It may help enhance focus, concentration, and cognitive performance, particularly during periods of stress or fatigue.

Incorporating Maca into Your Diet

Maca Powder: Maca powder is a versatile and convenient way to incorporate this superfood into your diet. Add it to smoothies, yogurt, oatmeal, or baked goods for an energizing boost.

Maca Capsules: Maca capsules or tablets provide a convenient option for those who prefer a more concentrated and standardized form of maca. Follow dosage recommendations and consult with a healthcare professional if needed.

Maca Tea: Maca tea can be made by steeping dried maca root slices or powder in hot water. Enjoy it alone or blend it with other herbs for added flavor and benefits.

Safety Considerations

Maca is generally considered safe for most people when consumed in recommended doses.

However, individuals with thyroid disorders or hormone-sensitive conditions should use caution when using maca, as it may affect hormone levels. Pregnant or breastfeeding women should consult with a healthcare professional before using maca supplements.

Maca root, with its rich nutritional profile and myriad health benefits, offers a natural and sustainable solution for promoting vitality, stamina, and hormonal balance. By incorporating maca into your daily routine, whether through powder, capsules, or tea, you can harness its energizing and rejuvenating properties, supporting your body, mind, and spirit on the journey to optimal health and vitality. With each serving, each sip, you embrace the power of nature's superfood, unlocking your full potential and embracing life with vigor and vitality.

Beetroot: The Vibrant Root of Health and Vitality

Beetroot (Beta vulgaris)

Introduction

Beneath its unassuming exterior, beetroot harbors a wealth of health-promoting properties, making it a versatile and valuable addition to any diet. With its vibrant hue and earthy flavor, beetroot not only adds color and depth to culinary creations but also offers a myriad of health benefits, ranging from cardiovascular support to athletic performance enhancement. In this exploration, we uncover the secrets of beetroot and its role as a powerhouse of nutrition and vitality.

Nutritional Profile

Beetroot is packed with essential nutrients, including vitamins, minerals, antioxidants, and dietary fiber, that contribute to its health-promoting properties. It is particularly rich in folate, manganese, potassium, and vitamin C, as well as betalains, a unique class of antioxidants found exclusively in beets.

Health Benefits of Beetroot

Cardiovascular Health: Beetroot is renowned for its cardiovascular benefits, thanks to its high nitrate content. Nitric oxide, produced from dietary nitrates, helps dilate blood vessels, improve blood flow, and lower blood pressure, reducing the risk of heart disease and stroke.

Exercise Performance: Beetroot juice has gained popularity as a natural sports supplement due to its potential to enhance exercise performance. Nitric oxide derived from dietary nitrates may improve oxygen utilization, increase endurance, and delay fatigue during physical activity, particularly endurance exercises like running and cycling.

Anti-Inflammatory Properties: Betalains, the pigments responsible for beetroot's vibrant color, possess potent anti-inflammatory properties. They help reduce inflammation, alleviate oxidative stress, and support joint health, making beetroot a valuable ally in the fight against chronic inflammation and related conditions.

Digestive Health: Beetroot is rich in dietary fiber, which promotes digestive regularity, supports gut health, and aids in weight management. Fiber adds bulk to stool, prevents constipation, and feeds beneficial gut bacteria, contributing to overall digestive wellness.

Liver Detoxification: Compounds in beetroot, such as betaine and antioxidants, support liver health and detoxification. They help protect liver cells from damage, promote bile production, and enhance the elimination of toxins and waste products from the body.

Incorporating Beetroot into Your Diet

Raw: Enjoy beetroot raw in salads or as a colorful addition to vegetable platters. Grate it, spiralize it, or thinly slice it for a crunchy and refreshing taste.

Cooked: Roast, steam, or boil beetroot for a tender and earthy addition to soups, stews, and side dishes. Its natural sweetness intensifies when cooked, adding depth of flavor to savory dishes.

Juiced: Extract the vibrant juice from beetroot and enjoy it on its own or blended with other fruits and vegetables for a nutrient-packed beverage. Add a splash of lemon or ginger for extra flavor.

Safety Considerations

While beetroot is generally safe for most people when consumed in moderate amounts, its rich pigment may cause harmless but noticeable changes in urine and stool color. Individuals with kidney stones or oxalate-related conditions should consume beetroot in moderation due to its oxalate content.

Beetroot, with its vibrant color and myriad health benefits, emerges as a true superfood for vitality and well-being. By incorporating beetroot into your diet on a regular basis, whether raw, cooked, or juiced, you can harness its nutritional power and support cardiovascular health, exercise performance, digestive wellness, and overall vitality. With each bite, each sip, you nourish your body, invigorate your senses, and embrace the abundance of nature's vibrant bounty.

Cordyceps: Nature's Secret to Vitality and Endurance

Cordyceps (Cordyceps sinensis)

Introduction

High in the misty mountains of Tibet and other regions of Asia, cordyceps mushrooms have long been revered for their remarkable health-promoting properties. Often referred to as the "caterpillar fungus" due to its unique life cycle, cordyceps is renowned for its ability to enhance vitality, endurance, and overall well-being. In this exploration, we uncover the secrets of cordyceps and its role as nature's secret to vitality and endurance.

Nutritional Profile

Cordyceps mushrooms are rich in bioactive compounds, including polysaccharides, nucleosides, peptides, and sterols, that contribute to their health-promoting properties. They are also a source of essential amino acids, vitamins, and minerals, making them a valuable addition to any diet.

Health Benefits of Cordyceps

Enhanced Energy and Endurance: Cordyceps is prized for its ability to increase energy levels, enhance endurance, and improve physical performance. It helps optimize oxygen utilization, increase ATP production, and reduce fatigue, making it a popular choice among athletes and active individuals.

Adaptogenic Properties: Cordyceps is classified as an adaptogen, a special class of herbs that help the body adapt to stress and restore balance. It helps regulate stress hormone levels, promote resilience to physical and emotional stressors, and support overall well-being.

Respiratory Health: Cordyceps has a long history of use in traditional Chinese medicine for respiratory conditions such as asthma, bronchitis, and coughs. It helps support lung function, reduce inflammation, and enhance respiratory endurance, making it beneficial for individuals with respiratory issues.

Immune Support: Cordyceps contains compounds, such as beta-glucans and cordycepin, that support immune function and enhance resistance to infections. It helps strengthen the body's natural defenses, promote immune balance, and support overall immune health.

Anti-Aging Properties: Cordyceps is revered for its anti-aging properties, which are attributed to its antioxidant and anti-inflammatory effects. It helps reduce oxidative stress, combat free radicals, and protect against age-related decline, promoting vitality and longevity.

Incorporating Cordyceps into Your Routine

Cordyceps Supplements: Cordyceps supplements, available in various forms such as capsules, tablets, and powders, provide a convenient way to incorporate this medicinal mushroom into your daily routine. Follow dosage recommendations and choose high-quality products from reputable brands.

Cordyceps Tea: Cordyceps tea can be made by steeping dried cordyceps mushrooms or cordyceps tea bags in hot water. Enjoy it alone or blend it with other herbs for added flavor and benefits.

Culinary Uses: Cordyceps mushrooms can be added to soups, stews, stir-fries, and other savory dishes for a nutritious and flavorful boost. They pair well with ingredients like garlic, ginger, mushrooms, and vegetables.

Safety Considerations

Cordyceps is generally safe for most people when consumed in recommended doses. However, individuals with autoimmune diseases or bleeding disorders should use caution when using cordyceps supplements. Pregnant or breastfeeding women should consult with a healthcare professional before using cordyceps.

Cordyceps mushrooms, with their potent health-promoting properties and centuries-old legacy, offer a natural and sustainable solution for enhancing vitality, endurance, and overall well-being. By incorporating cordyceps into your daily routine, whether through supplements, teas, or culinary creations, you can harness the power of nature's secret to vitality and endurance, supporting your body, mind, and spirit on the journey to optimal health and vitality. With each dose, each sip, each bite, you embrace the abundance of nature's timeless wisdom, unlocking your full potential and embracing life with vigor and vitality.

Herbal Remedies for Brighter Eyes and Clearer Vision

Introduction

Eyes are the windows to the soul, and caring for them is essential for overall well-being. While modern medicine offers many solutions for eye health, herbal remedies have been used for centuries to support and maintain optimal vision. In this exploration, we uncover the secrets of herbal remedies for eye health, offering natural solutions to enhance brightness, clarity, and vitality.

Nutritional Support for Eyes

Before delving into specific herbs, it's important to recognize the role of nutrition in maintaining eye health. Foods rich in vitamins A, C, and E, as well as antioxidants like lutein and zeaxanthin, play crucial roles in supporting eye function and protecting against age-related macular degeneration (AMD) and cataracts. Incorporating colorful fruits and vegetables, leafy greens, and omega-3 fatty acids into your diet can provide essential nutrients for optimal eye health.

Herbal Remedies for Eye Health

1. Bilberry (Vaccinium myrtillus): Bilberry is renowned for its vision-enhancing properties. Rich in anthocyanins and antioxidants, bilberry helps improve circulation to the eyes, protect against oxidative damage, and support night vision. It may also help reduce eye strain and fatigue, making it a valuable ally for those who spend long hours in front of screens.

2. Ginkgo (Ginkgo biloba): Ginkgo is prized for its ability to improve blood flow and circulation throughout the body, including to the eyes and brain. By enhancing circulation to the retina, ginkgo may help reduce the risk of age-related vision loss and support overall eye health. It also has antioxidant properties that protect against oxidative stress and inflammation.

3. Eyebright (Euphrasia officinalis): As its name suggests, eyebright has been traditionally used to support eye health and clarity. It contains compounds that help reduce inflammation, soothe irritated eyes, and alleviate symptoms of eye strain and allergies. Eyebright is often used in herbal eye washes and compresses to refresh and revitalize tired eyes.

4. Marigold (Tagetes erecta): Marigold, also known as calendula, is prized for its anti-inflammatory and antimicrobial properties. It contains lutein and zeaxanthin, two antioxidants that accumulate in the retina and help protect against oxidative damage from blue light and UV radiation. Marigold extracts may help reduce the risk of cataracts and AMD while promoting overall eye health.

5. Green Tea (Camellia sinensis): Green tea is rich in antioxidants called catechins, which have been shown to protect against oxidative stress and inflammation in the eyes. Regular consumption of green tea may help reduce the risk of glaucoma, diabetic retinopathy, and other eye conditions by supporting blood vessel health and reducing intraocular pressure.

Incorporating Herbal Remedies into Your Routine

Herbal remedies for eye health can be consumed in various forms, including teas, tinctures, capsules, and extracts. Additionally, some herbs can be used externally as eye washes, compresses, or poultices for targeted relief. When using herbal remedies, it's important to follow dosage recommendations and consult with a healthcare professional, especially if you have underlying health conditions or are taking medications.

Herbal remedies offer natural and holistic solutions for supporting and maintaining optimal eye health. By incorporating herbs like bilberry, ginkgo, eyebright, marigold, and green tea into your daily routine, you can nourish and protect your eyes, enhancing brightness, clarity, and vitality for years to come. With each sip of herbal tea, each application of herbal compress, you honor the wisdom of nature's pharmacy, nurturing your eyes and embracing the beauty of the world with clarity and grace.

Bilberry: Nature's Vision Booster

Bilberry (Vaccinium myrtillus)

Introduction

Nestled in the cool forests of Europe and North America, bilberry has long been revered for its remarkable vision-enhancing properties. With its deep blue-black berries and rich anthocyanin content, bilberry stands as a symbol of clarity, vitality, and eye health. In this exploration, we uncover the secrets of bilberry and its role as nature's vision booster.

Nutritional Profile

Bilberry is rich in bioactive compounds, including anthocyanins, flavonoids, and phenolic acids, that contribute to its health-promoting properties. These potent antioxidants help protect the eyes from oxidative damage, reduce inflammation, and support overall eye health. Bilberry also contains vitamins C and E, as well as essential minerals like manganese and potassium.

Health Benefits of Bilberry

Vision Enhancement: Bilberry is renowned for its ability to improve night vision and visual acuity. Anthocyanins in bilberry help enhance blood flow to the retina, strengthen capillaries, and protect against oxidative damage, promoting clarity and sharpness of vision, particularly in low-light conditions.

Eye Health Support: Bilberry's antioxidant properties help protect the eyes from age-related conditions such as macular degeneration and cataracts. Regular consumption of bilberry may help reduce the risk of vision loss, slow the progression of degenerative eye diseases, and support overall eye health.

Anti-Inflammatory Effects: Bilberry contains compounds that help reduce inflammation in the eyes and throughout the body. By inhibiting inflammatory pathways, bilberry may help alleviate symptoms of eye strain, fatigue, and irritation, promoting comfort and well-being.

Blood Sugar Regulation: Some studies suggest that bilberry may help regulate blood sugar levels and improve insulin sensitivity, which can benefit individuals with diabetes or metabolic syndrome. By supporting blood vessel health and reducing oxidative stress, bilberry may help prevent diabetic retinopathy and other complications associated with diabetes.

Cardiovascular Support: The antioxidant-rich nature of bilberry extends to cardiovascular health, where it helps protect against heart disease, hypertension, and atherosclerosis. By improving blood flow, reducing inflammation, and lowering cholesterol levels, bilberry supports heart health and overall vitality.

Incorporating Bilberry into Your Routine

Bilberry Supplements: Bilberry supplements are available in various forms, including capsules, tablets, and extracts. Choose high-quality products from reputable brands and follow dosage recommendations for optimal results.

Bilberry Tea: Bilberry tea can be made by steeping dried bilberry berries or bilberry tea bags in hot water. Enjoy it alone or blend it with other herbs for added flavor and benefits.

Culinary Uses: Fresh or dried bilberry berries can be added to smoothies, yogurt, oatmeal, or baked goods for a nutritious and delicious boost. Their sweet-tart flavor pairs well with a variety of foods and recipes.

Safety Considerations

Bilberry is generally safe for most people when consumed in recommended doses. However, individuals with bleeding disorders or those taking blood-thinning medications should use caution when using bilberry supplements, as it may increase the risk of bleeding. Pregnant or breastfeeding women should consult with a healthcare professional before using bilberry.

Bilberry, with its potent antioxidants and vision-enhancing properties, offers a natural and effective solution for supporting eye health and clarity. By incorporating bilberry into your daily routine, whether through supplements, tea, or culinary creations, you can nourish and protect your eyes, enhancing brightness, sharpness, and vitality for years to come. With each dose, each sip, each bite, you honor the wisdom of nature's bounty, embracing the beauty of the world with clarity and grace.

Eyebright: Nature's Soothing Solution for Clear Vision

Eyebright (Euphrasia officinalis)

Introduction

In the verdant meadows and grassy slopes of Europe, Eyebright blooms with delicate beauty, offering a gentle yet powerful remedy for tired and irritated eyes. Revered for centuries for its soothing and clarifying properties, Eyebright stands as nature's solution for promoting clear vision and ocular comfort. In this exploration, we uncover the secrets of Eyebright and its role in nurturing eye health and vitality.

Nutritional Profile

Eyebright contains a variety of bioactive compounds, including flavonoids, tannins, and iridoid glycosides, which contribute to its therapeutic effects. These compounds possess anti-inflammatory, astringent, and antioxidant properties, making Eyebright a valuable ally for supporting eye health and comfort.

Health Benefits of Eyebright

Eye Irritation Relief: Eyebright has been traditionally used to alleviate symptoms of eye irritation, including itching, redness, and dryness. Its anti-inflammatory and astringent properties help soothe inflamed tissues, reduce swelling, and relieve discomfort, making it an effective remedy for various eye conditions.

Allergy Symptom Relief: For individuals prone to seasonal allergies or allergic conjunctivitis, Eyebright offers natural relief from itching, watering, and inflammation of the eyes. Its ability to reduce allergic responses and soothe irritated mucous membranes makes it a valuable herbal remedy for allergy-related eye symptoms.

Eye Strain Alleviation: In today's digital age, prolonged screen time can lead to eye strain and fatigue. Eyebright may help alleviate symptoms of eye strain by refreshing and rejuvenating tired eyes, reducing redness, and promoting relaxation. Its gentle astringent properties help tone and tighten the delicate tissues surrounding the eyes, restoring comfort and vitality.

Vision Support: While Eyebright is not a cure for vision problems, it may help support overall eye health and clarity. Its antioxidant properties help protect the eyes from oxidative damage, reduce the risk of age-related macular degeneration (AMD), and promote ocular wellness, contributing to clearer and sharper vision over time.

Incorporating Eyebright into Your Routine

Eyebright Tea: Eyebright tea can be made by steeping dried Eyebright herb in hot water for 5-10 minutes. Allow it to cool slightly before using it as an eye wash or applying it to closed eyelids with a clean cloth for soothing relief.

Eyebright Eye Drops: Commercially available Eyebright eye drops or eye washes can be used to rinse irritated eyes and alleviate discomfort caused by allergies, dryness, or eye strain. Follow the manufacturer's instructions for proper usage and dosage.

Safety Considerations

While Eyebright is considered safe for most people when used externally as an eye wash or compress, it is important to avoid getting Eyebright preparations into the eyes. If you experience persistent or severe eye symptoms, consult with a healthcare professional for proper diagnosis and treatment.

Eyebright, with its gentle yet potent healing properties, offers a natural and effective solution for promoting clear vision and ocular comfort. By incorporating Eyebright into your eye care routine, whether through herbal teas, eye washes, or compresses, you can soothe irritation, alleviate discomfort, and support overall eye health with nature's gentle touch. With each application, each infusion, you honor the wisdom of nature's pharmacy, embracing the clarity and vitality of your precious gift of sight.

Ginkgo Biloba: Nature's Memory Enhancer and Circulation Booster

Ginkgo biloba

Introduction

In the shaded groves of Asia, the Ginkgo biloba tree stands as a living fossil, revered for its remarkable health benefits and longevity. For centuries, traditional healers have harnessed the power of Ginkgo biloba to enhance memory, improve circulation, and support overall well-being. In this exploration, we uncover the secrets of Ginkgo biloba and its role as nature's memory enhancer and circulation booster.

Nutritional Profile

Ginkgo biloba leaves contain a unique combination of bioactive compounds, including flavonoids, terpenoids, and ginkgolides, which contribute to its therapeutic effects. These compounds possess antioxidant, anti-inflammatory, and neuroprotective properties, making Ginkgo biloba a valuable ally for brain health and cognitive function.

Health Benefits of Ginkgo Biloba

Memory Enhancement: Ginkgo biloba is perhaps best known for its ability to enhance memory and cognitive function. By improving blood flow to the brain and increasing oxygen delivery to brain cells, Ginkgo biloba may help enhance mental clarity, focus, and memory recall, particularly in older adults experiencing age-related cognitive decline.

Improved Circulation: Ginkgo biloba is renowned for its vasodilatory effects, which help improve circulation throughout the body, including to the brain, heart, and extremities. By dilating blood vessels and reducing platelet aggregation, Ginkgo biloba may help reduce the risk of cardiovascular disease, peripheral artery disease, and related complications.

Antioxidant Protection: Ginkgo biloba is rich in antioxidants, which help protect cells from oxidative damage caused by free radicals. By neutralizing harmful molecules and reducing oxidative stress, Ginkgo biloba may help slow the aging process, support immune function, and reduce the risk of chronic diseases such as cancer and neurodegenerative disorders.

Eye Health Support: Ginkgo biloba's ability to improve circulation extends to the eyes, where it may help protect against age-related macular degeneration (AMD) and glaucoma. By enhancing blood flow to the retina and optic nerve, Ginkgo biloba supports ocular health and visual function, promoting clarity and vitality of vision.

Incorporating Ginkgo Biloba into Your Routine

Supplements: Ginkgo biloba supplements are available in various forms, including capsules, tablets, and liquid extracts. Choose standardized extracts containing a specific concentration of ginkgo flavonoids and terpenoids for optimal potency and effectiveness.

Tea: Ginkgo biloba tea can be made by steeping dried ginkgo leaves in hot water for 5-10 minutes. Enjoy it alone or blend it with other herbs for added flavor and benefits. Note that ginkgo tea may have a slightly bitter taste.

Safety Considerations

While Ginkgo biloba is generally safe for most people when taken in recommended doses, it may interact with certain medications, including blood thinners, antidepressants, and anticonvulsants. Pregnant or breastfeeding women, as well as individuals with bleeding disorders or seizure disorders, should consult with a healthcare professional before using Ginkgo biloba supplements.

Ginkgo biloba, with its potent memory-enhancing and circulation-boosting properties, offers a natural and effective solution for supporting brain health, cardiovascular function, and overall well-being. By incorporating Ginkgo biloba into your daily routine, whether through supplements or herbal teas, you can nourish and protect your mind, body, and spirit with nature's timeless wisdom. With each dose, each sip, each breath, you honor the resilience and vitality of your precious gift of life.

Saffron: The Golden Spice of Health and Culinary Delight

Saffron (Crocus sativus)

Introduction

In the sun-drenched fields of Mediterranean regions, saffron blooms as a symbol of luxury, flavor, and wellness. Renowned for its vibrant color, distinctive aroma, and myriad health benefits, saffron stands as a prized spice with a rich history of culinary and medicinal use. In this exploration, we uncover the secrets of saffron and its role as nature's golden spice of health and culinary delight.

Nutritional Profile

Saffron derives its characteristic color, flavor, and aroma from its bioactive compounds, including crocin, picrocrocin, and safranal. These compounds possess antioxidant, anti-inflammatory, and neuroprotective properties, making saffron a valuable addition to both culinary and medicinal preparations.

Health Benefits of Saffron

Mood Enhancement: Saffron has been traditionally used as a natural remedy for mood disorders such as depression and anxiety. Compounds in saffron, particularly safranal, may help regulate neurotransmitter levels in the brain, promote relaxation, and alleviate symptoms of stress and mood swings.

Antioxidant Protection: Saffron is rich in antioxidants, which help neutralize free radicals and reduce oxidative stress in the body. By protecting cells from damage caused by environmental toxins and aging, saffron may help prevent chronic diseases such as cancer, heart disease, and neurodegenerative disorders.

Eye Health Support: Saffron contains compounds that benefit eye health by protecting against age-related macular degeneration (AMD) and cataracts. Crocin, a key component of saffron, helps improve blood flow to the retina, reduce inflammation, and protect against oxidative damage, promoting clarity and vitality of vision.

Brain Health and Cognitive Function: Saffron has been shown to support brain health and cognitive function by enhancing memory, learning, and neuroplasticity. Compounds in saffron may help increase levels of brain-derived neurotrophic factor (BDNF), a protein that supports the growth and survival of brain cells, improving cognitive performance and reducing the risk of neurodegenerative diseases such as Alzheimer's.

Incorporating Saffron into Your Cuisine

Saffron Threads: Saffron threads can be infused in hot water or milk to extract their color, flavor, and aroma before adding them to dishes. Simply soak a few threads in warm liquid for 15-20 minutes, then use the infused liquid to flavor soups, stews, rice dishes, or desserts.

Saffron Powder: Saffron powder can be ground from dried saffron threads using a mortar and pestle or spice grinder. Add a pinch of saffron powder to recipes for a burst of color and flavor, or use it to make saffron-infused oils, sauces, or dressings.

Safety Considerations

While saffron is generally safe for culinary use, excessive consumption of saffron supplements may cause adverse effects such as nausea, vomiting, and dizziness. Pregnant or breastfeeding women should avoid high doses of saffron due to the risk of uterine contractions. Always use saffron in moderation and consult with a healthcare professional before using saffron supplements, especially if you have underlying health conditions or are taking medications.

Saffron, with its rich color, exquisite flavor, and myriad health benefits, offers a culinary and medicinal treasure trove for enhancing wellness and vitality. By incorporating saffron into your cuisine, whether as a spice, infusion, or supplement, you can savor its golden essence and nourish your body, mind, and spirit with nature's timeless wisdom. With each dish, each sip, each moment of indulgence, you honor the abundance and richness of life, embracing the joy and vitality that saffron brings to every meal.

Creating Your Herbal Medicine Cabinet

Building your own herbal medicine cabinet is like curating a toolkit for natural health and wellness. By having a selection of essential herbs on hand, you empower yourself to address minor ailments and support overall well-being. Here’s how you can create your own herbal medicine cabinet:

Essential Herbs to Keep at Home

1. Chamomile (Matricaria chamomilla):
   - Known for its calming properties, chamomile is excellent for soothing digestive issues, promoting relaxation, and relieving anxiety.

2. Echinacea (Echinacea purpurea):
   - A powerful immune booster, echinacea helps to prevent and shorten the duration of colds and flu. It stimulates the production of white blood cells, enhancing the body's defense mechanisms.

3. Ginger (Zingiber officinale):
   - Ginger is a versatile herb with anti-inflammatory and digestive benefits. It alleviates nausea, supports digestion, and reduces muscle pain and inflammation.

4. Peppermint (Mentha piperita):
   - Peppermint is cooling and refreshing, making it ideal for relieving digestive discomfort, headaches, and respiratory congestion. It also acts as a natural energy booster.

5. Lavender (Lavandula angustifolia):
   - Lavender is renowned for its calming and sedative effects. It promotes relaxation, reduces anxiety, aids in sleep, and soothes skin irritations.

6. Calendula (Calendula officinalis):
   - Calendula is a gentle yet effective herb for skin healing. It has anti-inflammatory and antimicrobial properties, making it ideal for treating cuts, wounds, rashes, and minor burns.

7. Nettles (Urtica dioica):
   - Nettles are rich in vitamins and minerals, making them a nourishing tonic for overall health. They are particularly beneficial for allergies, hay fever, and respiratory conditions.

8. Garlic (Allium sativum):
   - Garlic is a potent antimicrobial and immune enhancer. It supports cardiovascular health, lowers blood pressure and cholesterol, and helps fight infections.

Growing and Harvesting Your Own Herbs

If space allows, consider growing your own herbs. This ensures a fresh and sustainable supply while connecting you with nature's healing power. Choose a sunny spot in your garden or balcony and select herbs that thrive in your climate. Some easy-to-grow options include basil, mint, thyme, and sage. Remember to harvest herbs in the morning when their essential oils are most potent, and dry them thoroughly before storing.

Making Your Own Herbal Preparations

Experiment with different herbal preparations to find what works best for you. Common methods include:

- Herbal Teas: Steep dried herbs in hot water to make soothing teas.
- Tinctures: Extract herbs in alcohol or glycerin to create potent liquid extracts.
- Infused Oils: Infuse herbs in carrier oils like olive or coconut oil for topical use.
- Salves and Balms: Combine infused oils with beeswax to make healing salves for skin conditions.

Storing and Preserving Herbs

Proper storage is essential to maintain the potency and freshness of your herbs. Store dried herbs in airtight containers away from heat, light, and moisture. Label containers with the herb name and date of harvest or purchase. Keep tinctures and infused oils in dark glass bottles to protect them from light degradation. Check for signs of spoilage regularly and discard any herbs that appear moldy or discolored.

By curating your herbal medicine cabinet and learning how to use these powerful botanicals, you can take charge of your health naturally and effectively. Remember to consult with a healthcare professional or herbalist for personalized advice and guidance.

Essential Herbs to Keep at Home

Building your herbal medicine cabinet starts with selecting a few key herbs that can address a variety of common health concerns. These essential herbs are versatile, safe, and effective, making them must-haves for any home apothecary. Here are some of the top herbs to keep at home:

1. Chamomile (Matricaria chamomilla):
   - Properties: Calming, anti-inflammatory, digestive.
   - Uses: Chamomile is renowned for its calming effects, making it an excellent remedy for stress, anxiety, and insomnia. It also soothes digestive discomfort, including indigestion, gas, and bloating.

2. Echinacea (Echinacea purpurea):
   - Properties: Immune-boosting, anti-inflammatory, antimicrobial.
   - Uses: Echinacea is a powerful immune stimulant that can help prevent and shorten the duration of colds, flu, and other infections. It stimulates the body's natural defense mechanisms and reduces inflammation.

3. Ginger (Zingiber officinale):
   - Properties: Warming, anti-inflammatory, digestive.
   - Uses: Ginger is a versatile herb with a wide range of health benefits. It aids digestion, relieves nausea and motion sickness, reduces inflammation and muscle pain, and boosts circulation.

4. Peppermint (Mentha piperita):
   - Properties: Cooling, digestive, analgesic.
   - Uses: Peppermint is known for its cooling and refreshing properties. It soothes digestive discomfort, including indigestion, gas, and bloating. It also relieves headaches, muscle tension, and respiratory congestion.

5. Lavender (Lavandula angustifolia):
- Properties: Calming, sedative, antimicrobial.
- Uses: Lavender is prized for its calming and sedative effects, making it a popular remedy for stress, anxiety, and insomnia. It also has antimicrobial properties and can soothe skin irritations and minor burns.

6. Calendula (Calendula officinalis):
- Properties: Healing, anti-inflammatory, antimicrobial.
- Uses: Calendula is a gentle yet effective herb for skin health. It promotes wound healing, reduces inflammation, and has antimicrobial properties. It's commonly used to treat cuts, scrapes, rashes, and minor burns.

7. Nettles (Urtica dioica):
- Properties: Nutritive, anti-inflammatory, diuretic.
- Uses: Nettles are highly nutritious and support overall health and vitality. They are particularly beneficial for allergies, hay fever, and respiratory conditions due to their anti-inflammatory and antihistamine properties.

8. Garlic (Allium sativum):
- Properties: Antimicrobial, immune-boosting, cardiovascular.
- Uses: Garlic is a potent antimicrobial herb that can help fight infections, including colds, flu, and fungal infections. It also supports cardiovascular health by lowering blood pressure and cholesterol levels.

By keeping these essential herbs on hand, you'll have natural remedies readily available to address a wide range of health issues. Whether you prefer to use them in teas, tinctures, or topical preparations, these versatile herbs are invaluable allies for maintaining health and well-being.

Growing and Harvesting Your Own Herbs

Growing your own herbs is not only rewarding but also ensures a fresh and sustainable supply of medicinal plants for your herbal medicine cabinet. Whether you have a spacious garden or a small balcony, you can cultivate a variety of herbs that thrive in your climate and growing conditions. Here's a guide to growing and harvesting your own herbs:

Choosing the Right Herbs

1. Assess Your Space: Determine how much space you have available for growing herbs. Consider factors such as sunlight, water access, and climate conditions.

2. Select Herbs: Choose herbs that are well-suited to your growing environment. Some herbs, like basil and mint, prefer full sun, while others, like parsley and cilantro, can tolerate partial shade.

3. Start Small: If you're new to gardening, start with a few easy-to-grow herbs, such as basil, thyme, and rosemary. As you gain experience, you can expand your herb garden and try growing more challenging varieties.

Planting Herbs

1. Choose Containers or Beds: Herbs can be grown in containers, raised beds, or directly in the ground. Make sure containers have drainage holes to prevent waterlogging.

2. Use Quality Soil: Use well-draining soil with plenty of organic matter for optimal herb growth. You can amend the soil with compost or aged manure to improve fertility.

3. Watering: Herbs generally prefer moderate watering. Water them deeply when the top inch of soil feels dry to the touch, but avoid overwatering, as this can lead to root rot.

4. Maintenance: Regularly remove weeds, dead leaves, and spent flowers to promote healthy growth. Prune herbs regularly to encourage bushier growth and prevent them from becoming leggy.

Harvesting Herbs

1. Timing: Harvest herbs in the morning when their essential oils are most concentrated. Avoid harvesting during the hottest part of the day, as this can cause wilting.

2. Method: Use sharp scissors or pruning shears to harvest herbs. Cut stems above a leaf node to encourage new growth. For leafy herbs like basil and parsley, pinch off individual leaves as needed.

3. Frequency: Harvest herbs regularly to encourage continuous growth. Avoid harvesting more than one-third of the plant at a time, as this can stress the plant.

4. Drying Herbs: To preserve herbs for future use, you can dry them by hanging bundles upside down in a well-ventilated area away from direct sunlight. Once dry, store the herbs in airtight containers away from heat and moisture.

5. Freezing Herbs: Alternatively, you can freeze fresh herbs by chopping them finely and placing them in ice cube trays filled with water or olive oil. Once frozen, transfer the herb cubes to a freezer bag for long-term storage.

Common Herbs to Grow

- Basil: Aromatic herb used in cooking and teas.
- Mint: Refreshing herb with digestive and respiratory benefits.
- Rosemary: Fragrant herb with antioxidant and anti-inflammatory properties.
- Thyme: Versatile herb with antimicrobial and expectorant properties.
- Parsley: Nutritious herb rich in vitamins and minerals.
- Lavender: Calming herb used in aromatherapy and herbal preparations.

By growing and harvesting your own herbs, you can enjoy a sustainable and bountiful supply of medicinal plants right at your fingertips. Experiment with different varieties, and don't be afraid to get your hands dirty in the garden!

Making Your Own Herbal Preparations

Harnessing the healing power of herbs is not only cost-effective but also empowering. By making your own herbal preparations, you can customize remedies to suit your specific needs and preferences. Whether you prefer teas, tinctures, salves, or oils, here's how you can create your own herbal remedies at home:

Herbal Teas

1. Selecting Herbs: Choose dried herbs or herbal blends that suit your desired outcome. For

example, chamomile and lavender are calming herbs, while ginger and peppermint are digestive aids.

2. Brewing: Place 1-2 teaspoons of dried herbs per cup of hot water in a teapot or mug. Cover and steep for 5-10 minutes, depending on the strength desired.

3. Straining: Once steeped, strain the tea using a fine-mesh sieve or tea strainer to remove the herbs. Sweeten with honey or add lemon, if desired.

4. Storing: Drink herbal tea immediately for maximum freshness. Leftover tea can be stored in the refrigerator for up to 24 hours.

Herbal Tinctures

1. Choosing Herbs: Select dried herbs with medicinal properties suited to your needs. Common choices include echinacea for immune support, and valerian for relaxation.

2. Alcohol Extraction: Place dried herbs in a clean glass jar and cover with alcohol such as vodka or brandy. Ensure the herbs are completely submerged.

3. Maceration: Seal the jar tightly and store it in a cool, dark place for 4-6 weeks, shaking daily to agitate the mixture.

4. Straining and Bottling: After maceration, strain the tincture through cheesecloth or a fine-mesh sieve to remove the plant material. Transfer the liquid to amber glass dropper bottles for storage.

5. Dosage: To use, dilute the tincture in water or juice according to dosage instructions. Typically, 1-2 dropperfuls (30-60 drops) are taken up to three times per day.

Herbal Salves and Balms

1. Infused Oil: Start by infusing dried herbs in a carrier oil such as olive oil or coconut oil. Place the herbs in a clean glass jar and cover with oil. Seal the jar and place it in a sunny windowsill for 2-4 weeks, shaking daily.

2. Straining: After infusion, strain the oil through cheesecloth or a fine-mesh sieve to remove the plant material. Squeeze out any excess oil from the herbs.

3. Beeswax Melt: In a double boiler, melt beeswax over low heat. Once melted, add the infused oil and stir until well combined. The ratio of oil to beeswax depends on the desired consistency.

4. Cooling and Storing: Pour the mixture into clean, sterilized jars or tins and allow it to cool completely before sealing. Store salves in a cool, dark place away from direct sunlight.

Herbal Infused Oils

1. Selecting Herbs: Choose dried herbs with medicinal properties suited to your needs. Common choices include calendula for skin healing, and arnica for muscle pain relief.

2. Infusion: Place the herbs in a clean glass jar and cover with a carrier oil such as olive oil or sweet almond oil. Ensure the herbs are completely submerged.

3. Solar Infusion: Seal the jar tightly and place it in a sunny windowsill for 2-4 weeks, shaking daily to agitate the mixture.

4. Straining: After infusion, strain the oil through cheesecloth or a fine-mesh sieve to remove the plant material. Squeeze out any excess oil from the herbs.

5. Bottling: Transfer the infused oil to clean, sterilized glass bottles or jars for storage. Label the bottles with the herb used and the date of preparation.

By making your own herbal preparations, you can take control of your health and well-being while connecting more deeply with the natural world. Experiment with different herbs and formulations to find what works best for you, and remember to always label your creations for safety and future reference.

Storing and Preserving Herbs

Proper storage is essential for maintaining the potency and freshness of your herbs, whether they are freshly harvested or purchased. By following these guidelines, you can ensure that your herbs remain vibrant and flavorful for longer periods:

Drying Herbs

1. Air Drying: Hang fresh herbs upside down in small bundles in a well-ventilated area away from direct sunlight. Ensure that the herbs are completely dry before storing.

2. Dehydrator: Use a food dehydrator to dry herbs quickly and efficiently. Spread the herbs in a single layer on the dehydrator trays and follow the manufacturer's instructions for drying times.

3. Oven Drying: Place herbs on a baking sheet lined with parchment paper and dry them in a preheated oven set to the lowest temperature (usually around 100°F or 40°C). Keep the oven door slightly ajar to allow moisture to escape.

4. Microwave Drying: Microwave small batches of herbs on a microwave-safe plate lined with paper towels. Microwave on high for 1-2 minutes, checking every 30 seconds until the herbs are dry.

Storing Dried Herbs

1. Airtight Containers: Store dried herbs in clean, airtight containers such as glass jars or resealable plastic bags. Make sure the containers are completely dry to prevent mold and spoilage.

2. Cool, Dark Place: Keep dried herbs in a cool, dark place away from heat, light, and moisture. Avoid storing them near the stove or in direct sunlight, as this can degrade their flavor and potency.

3. Labeling: Label containers with the name of the herb and the date of harvest or purchase. This helps you keep track of the herbs and ensures you use them before they lose their potency.

4. Whole vs. Ground: Consider storing herbs in their whole form whenever possible, as they tend to retain their flavor and aroma longer than ground herbs. Grind or crush the herbs just before use for maximum flavor.

Freezing Herbs

1. Flash Freezing: Wash and dry fresh herbs thoroughly, then chop or mince them finely. Spread the chopped herbs in a single layer on a baking sheet lined with parchment paper and place it in the freezer until the herbs are frozen solid.

2. Storage Bags: Transfer the frozen herbs to labeled freezer bags or airtight containers for long-term storage. Remove as much air as possible from the bags before sealing to prevent freezer burn.

3. Usage: Frozen herbs can be added directly to soups, stews, sauces, and other cooked dishes without thawing. Alternatively, thaw them in the refrigerator before use for salads, garnishes, or other raw applications.

Using Preserved Herbs

1. Rehydration: If using dried herbs, rehydrate them by soaking them in warm water for 10-15 minutes before use. This helps release their essential oils and flavors.

2. Adjusting Quantities: Keep in mind that dried herbs are more concentrated than fresh herbs, so you may need to adjust the quantities in recipes accordingly. As a general rule, use about one-third to one-half the amount of dried herbs compared to fresh herbs.

3. Storage Check: Periodically check stored herbs for signs of spoilage, such as mold, discoloration, or off odors. Discard any herbs that show signs of deterioration to prevent contamination of the rest of your herbs.

By storing and preserving your herbs properly, you can extend their shelf life and ensure that you have a steady supply of flavorful and aromatic ingredients for your culinary creations and herbal remedies. Experiment with different preservation methods to find the ones that work best for your herbs and your cooking style.

Conclusion: Embracing a Holistic Lifestyle

In our journey through the world of herbal medicine, we've explored the rich tapestry of nature's remedies and learned how to harness the healing power of herbs to support our health and well-being. As we conclude our exploration, it's essential to reflect on the broader implications of herbalism and its role in promoting a holistic lifestyle.

Integrating Mind, Body, and Spirit

At its core, herbal medicine is about more than just treating symptoms; it's about nurturing the interconnectedness of mind, body, and spirit. By embracing herbal remedies, we honor the wisdom of traditional healing practices that recognize the profound connection between our physical health, emotional well-being, and spiritual vitality.

Cultivating Awareness and Connection

Herbalism invites us to cultivate a deeper awareness of ourselves and our environment. As we connect with the plants that nourish and heal us, we develop a greater appreciation for the natural world and our place within it. This connection fosters a sense of stewardship and reverence for the Earth, inspiring us to live in harmony with the rhythms of nature.

Empowering Self-Care and Wellness

One of the most empowering aspects of herbal medicine is its emphasis on self-care and wellness. By learning how to grow, harvest, and prepare our own herbal remedies, we reclaim agency over our health and reduce our reliance on external interventions. Herbalism empowers us to take proactive steps towards prevention and wellness, rather than simply reacting to illness.

Embracing Diversity and Individuality

Just as every plant in nature is unique, so too is every individual. Herbal medicine celebrates this diversity and honors the uniqueness of each person's body and experiences. There is no one-size-fits-all approach in herbalism; instead, we are encouraged to listen to our bodies, trust our intuition, and adapt our herbal practices to meet our individual needs.

Fostering Community and Connection

Herbalism has a long history of being passed down through generations within communities. In today's world, it offers us an opportunity to reconnect with our roots and forge meaningful connections with others who share our passion for natural healing. Whether through herbal workshops, gardening groups, or online forums, herbalism brings people together in a shared pursuit of health and vitality.

Embracing a Sustainable Future

As we look to the future, herbalism offers a vision of health care that is sustainable, accessible, and rooted in the wisdom of the past. By embracing herbal remedies and incorporating them into our daily lives, we not only support our own well-being but also contribute to the health of our planet. Herbalism reminds us that true healing begins with a deep respect for the Earth and all of its inhabitants.

In closing, let us carry forward the lessons of herbal medicine with gratitude and reverence. May we continue to cultivate a holistic lifestyle that honors the interconnectedness of all things and fosters health, harmony, and vitality for ourselves and future generations.

Combining Herbs with Diet and Exercise

In our pursuit of holistic health and well-being, integrating herbal remedies with a balanced diet and regular exercise is paramount. By harmonizing these elements, we can optimize our physical, mental, and emotional vitality. Here's how to combine herbs with diet and exercise to create a comprehensive approach to wellness:

Herbal Support for Nutrition

1. Nutrient-Rich Herbs: Incorporate nutrient-rich herbs into your diet to enhance its nutritional value. Herbs like nettle, dandelion greens, and parsley are packed with vitamins, minerals, and antioxidants.

2. Herbal Supplements: Supplement your diet with herbal extracts or capsules to fill nutritional gaps. Herbs like spirulina, chlorella, and moringa provide concentrated doses of essential nutrients.

3. Herbal Teas: Enjoy herbal teas throughout the day as a nourishing beverage. Choose herbs like ginger, turmeric, and holy basil, which support digestion, reduce inflammation, and boost immunity.

Herbal Support for Exercise

1. Pre-Workout Herbs: Use energizing herbs to prepare for exercise and enhance performance. Herbs like ginseng, rhodiola, and maca increase stamina, improve endurance, and reduce fatigue.

2. Post-Workout Recovery: Support post-workout recovery with herbs that reduce inflammation and promote muscle repair. Herbs like turmeric, ginger, and boswellia help alleviate soreness and support tissue healing.

3. Adaptogenic Support: Incorporate adaptogenic herbs into your routine to help your body adapt to physical stress. Herbs like ashwagandha, eleuthero, and holy basil support adrenal health and balance cortisol levels.

Herbal Support for Weight Management

1. Metabolism-Boosting Herbs: Support metabolism and weight management with herbs that increase thermogenesis and fat burning. Herbs like green tea, cayenne pepper, and cinnamon enhance calorie expenditure and fat oxidation.

2. Appetite-Suppressing Herbs: Use herbs to help curb cravings and reduce appetite. Herbs like garcinia cambogia, yerba mate, and gymnema sylvestre help control hunger and promote satiety.

3. Digestive Support: Maintain digestive health to support weight management and overall well-being. Herbs like fennel, ginger, and peppermint aid digestion, reduce bloating, and alleviate gastrointestinal discomfort.

Integrating Herbal Remedies into Meals

1. Herbal Seasonings: Use fresh or dried herbs as seasonings in your meals to add flavor and enhance nutritional value. Experiment with different combinations of herbs to create delicious and healthful dishes.

2. Herbal Infusions: Infuse oils, vinegars, and dressings with herbs to incorporate their benefits into your meals. Herbs like rosemary, thyme, and oregano add depth of flavor and antioxidant protection.

3. Herbal Garnishes: Use fresh herbs as garnishes to add color, texture, and flavor to your dishes. Herbs like parsley, cilantro, and basil not only enhance the visual appeal of your meals but also provide a nutritional boost.

Mindful Eating and Herbal Support

1. Herbal Tea Rituals: Incorporate herbal tea rituals into your daily routine as a mindful practice. Take time to savor the aroma and flavor of your tea, and allow it to nourish and ground you.

2. Herbal Tonics: Create herbal tonics or elixirs to support specific health goals and cultivate a sense of well-being. Experiment with adaptogens, nervines, and tonic herbs to create personalized blends.

3. Herbal Mindfulness: Practice herbal mindfulness by connecting with the plants you consume. Reflect on the journey of the herbs from seed to cup or plate, and express gratitude for their healing gifts.

By combining herbs with a balanced diet and regular exercise, we can create a synergistic approach to health and wellness that nourishes our bodies, minds, and spirits. Let us embrace the wisdom of nature and cultivate vitality from the inside out.

The Role of Mindfulness and Stress Management

In our fast-paced modern world, stress has become a ubiquitous presence, taking a toll on our physical, mental, and emotional well-being. Mindfulness practices offer a powerful antidote to the chaos of everyday life, helping us cultivate inner peace, resilience, and balance. Here's how mindfulness and stress management play a crucial role in promoting holistic health:

Understanding Stress

1. Impact on Health: Chronic stress can wreak havoc on our bodies, contributing to a wide range of health problems, including heart disease, digestive issues, anxiety, and depression.

2. Mind-Body Connection: Stress not only affects us mentally and emotionally but also has tangible effects on our physiology, triggering the release of stress hormones like cortisol and adrenaline.

The Power of Mindfulness

1. Present Moment Awareness: Mindfulness involves paying attention to the present moment with openness, curiosity, and acceptance. By cultivating present moment awareness, we can break free from the grip of stress and anxiety.

2. Stress Reduction: Mindfulness practices, such as meditation, deep breathing, and body scans, have been shown to reduce stress levels and promote relaxation by activating the body's natural relaxation response.

Integrating Mindfulness into Daily Life

1. Mindful Eating: Practice mindful eating by paying attention to the flavors, textures, and sensations of each bite. Eating mindfully can help prevent overeating, improve digestion, and enhance our relationship with food.

2. Mindful Movement: Engage in mindful movement practices like yoga, tai chi, or qigong to cultivate awareness of the body and breath. These practices promote relaxation, flexibility, and balance.

Herbal Allies for Stress Management

1. Adaptogenic Herbs: Incorporate adaptogenic herbs like ashwagandha, holy basil, and rhodiola into your daily routine to support the body's response to stress. Adaptogens help increase resilience to stress and promote overall well-being.

2. Nervine Herbs: Nervine herbs like chamomile, lemon balm, and passionflower have calming and soothing properties that help reduce anxiety, promote relaxation, and support restful sleep.

Building a Mindfulness Practice

1. Start Small: Begin with short, manageable periods of mindfulness practice, such as 5-10 minutes of meditation or deep breathing exercises each day. Gradually increase the duration as you become

more comfortable.

2. Consistency is Key: Make mindfulness a regular part of your daily routine by scheduling time for practice and committing to it consistently. Set reminders on your phone or incorporate mindfulness into existing habits, such as brushing your teeth or taking a shower.

Stress Management Strategies

1. Self-Care Rituals: Prioritize self-care activities that nourish your body, mind, and soul, such as taking relaxing baths, spending time in nature, or engaging in creative pursuits.

2. Healthy Boundaries: Set boundaries to protect your time, energy, and emotional well-being. Learn to say no to commitments that drain you and prioritize activities that bring you joy and fulfillment.

The Mind-Body Connection

1. Stress Reduction Techniques: Practice stress reduction techniques like progressive muscle relaxation, guided imagery, or mindfulness-based stress reduction (MBSR) to promote relaxation and reduce stress-related symptoms.

2. Holistic Approach: Take a holistic approach to stress management by addressing the underlying causes of stress, including lifestyle factors, relationships, and environmental triggers. Explore how diet, exercise, sleep, and social support can influence your stress levels.

Cultivating Resilience

1. Mindful Resilience: Cultivate resilience by approaching life's challenges with mindfulness and compassion. Recognize that setbacks and obstacles are a natural part of the human experience and an opportunity for growth and learning.

2. Community Support: Seek support from friends, family, or support groups to share your experiences, gain perspective, and receive encouragement during difficult times. Remember, you are not alone on your journey.

Embracing Mindfulness as a Way of Life

1. Moment-to-Moment Awareness: Embrace mindfulness as a way of life by bringing awareness to every moment, whether you're eating, walking, working, or spending time with loved ones. Cultivate a sense of presence and aliveness in all that you do.

2. Non-Judgmental Awareness: Practice non-judgmental awareness by observing your thoughts, feelings, and sensations without attachment or aversion. Cultivate an attitude of curiosity, openness, and acceptance toward your inner experiences.

In conclusion, mindfulness and stress management are powerful tools for promoting holistic health and well-being. By integrating mindfulness practices into our daily lives and harnessing the healing power of herbs, we can cultivate inner peace, resilience, and vitality in the face of life's challenges. Let us embrace the present moment with mindfulness and compassion, knowing that true healing begins from within.

Building a Sustainable Approach to Health

In our pursuit of well-being, it's crucial to adopt a sustainable approach that nurtures not only our own health but also the health of the planet and future generations. By embracing holistic practices and mindful choices, we can create a lifestyle that promotes vitality, resilience, and harmony. Here's how to build a sustainable approach to health:

Honoring the Body

1. Nutrient-Rich Diet: Prioritize whole, unprocessed foods that nourish your body with essential vitamins, minerals, and antioxidants. Choose organic and locally sourced ingredients whenever possible to support both your health and the environment.

2. Hydration: Stay hydrated with clean, filtered water to support cellular function, digestion, and detoxification. Reduce waste by using reusable water bottles and investing in water filtration systems.

Embracing Movement and Exercise

1. Physical Activity: Incorporate regular movement and exercise into your daily routine to promote cardiovascular health, strength, flexibility, and mental well-being. Choose activities that you enjoy and that align with your interests and lifestyle.

2. Outdoor Activities: Take advantage of outdoor activities like hiking, biking, gardening, and swimming to connect with nature and reap the benefits of fresh air, sunlight, and natural surroundings.

Cultivating Mental and Emotional Well-Being

1. Mindfulness Practices: Engage in mindfulness practices such as meditation, deep breathing, and yoga to cultivate inner peace, resilience, and emotional balance. These practices help reduce stress, anxiety, and depression while promoting a sense of presence and clarity.

2. Stress Management: Develop effective stress management strategies to cope with life's challenges and setbacks. Prioritize self-care activities that nourish your mind, body, and spirit, such as journaling, spending time in nature, and seeking support from loved ones.

Prioritizing Sleep and Rest

1. Quality Sleep: Make sleep a priority by establishing a consistent sleep schedule and creating a relaxing bedtime routine. Create a sleep-friendly environment by minimizing noise, light, and electronic distractions in the bedroom.

2. Rest and Recovery: Allow time for rest and recovery to recharge your body and mind. Listen to your body's signals and honor its need for rest, relaxation, and downtime.

Connecting with Nature

1. Nature Therapy: Spend time in nature regularly to experience the healing benefits of the natural world. Engage in activities like forest bathing, nature walks, or outdoor picnics to reduce stress, boost mood, and enhance overall well-being.

2. Environmental Stewardship: Take steps to minimize your environmental footprint and protect the

planet for future generations. Reduce waste, conserve resources, and support sustainable practices in your daily life.

Integrating Herbal Medicine

1. Herbal Remedies: Incorporate herbal remedies into your health and wellness routine to support natural healing and vitality. Explore the diverse benefits of medicinal herbs for physical, mental, and emotional well-being.

2. Sustainable Practices: Source herbs ethically and sustainably to ensure their long-term availability and ecological integrity. Choose organic, wildcrafted, or locally grown herbs whenever possible, and support companies that prioritize sustainability and fair trade practices.

Building Resilience and Adaptability

1. Holistic Resilience: Cultivate resilience by adopting a holistic approach to health that addresses the interconnectedness of mind, body, and spirit. Embrace life's challenges as opportunities for growth, learning, and transformation.

2. Adaptive Strategies: Develop adaptive strategies to navigate uncertainty and change with grace and flexibility. Cultivate a growth mindset, cultivate self-awareness, and embrace the power of community and connection.

In conclusion, building a sustainable approach to health requires a commitment to holistic well-being, environmental stewardship, and mindful living. By honoring the body, embracing movement and exercise, cultivating mental and emotional well-being, prioritizing sleep and rest, connecting with nature, integrating herbal medicine, and building resilience and adaptability, we can create a lifestyle that promotes vitality, resilience, and harmony for ourselves and the planet. Let us embrace the journey toward sustainable health with intention, compassion, and a deep sense of reverence for the interconnectedness of all life.

Future Directions in Herbal Medicine

As we look ahead, the future of herbal medicine is filled with promise and potential. Advancements in scientific research, technological innovation, and integrative approaches are shaping the landscape of herbal medicine, paving the way for new discoveries, applications, and collaborations. Here are some future directions in herbal medicine:

Evidence-Based Research

1. Clinical Trials: Continued investment in rigorous clinical trials and research studies is essential for validating the safety, efficacy, and mechanisms of action of herbal remedies. This evidence-based approach will help integrate herbal medicine into mainstream healthcare and improve patient outcomes.

2. Bioavailability Studies: Research into the bioavailability and pharmacokinetics of herbal compounds will enhance our understanding of how herbs are absorbed, metabolized, and excreted in the body. This knowledge will inform dosage recommendations and optimize therapeutic outcomes.

Personalized Medicine

1. Genomic Medicine: Advances in genomic medicine and personalized diagnostics will enable healthcare providers to tailor herbal treatments to individual genetic profiles and metabolic pathways. This precision medicine approach holds promise for optimizing treatment outcomes and minimizing adverse reactions.

2. Biomarker Testing: Biomarker testing and functional medicine assessments will help identify underlying imbalances and root causes of disease, guiding the selection of targeted herbal interventions and therapeutic protocols.

Integrative Healthcare

1. Collaborative Care Models: Integration of herbal medicine into multidisciplinary healthcare teams will facilitate collaborative care models that combine conventional treatments with complementary and alternative therapies. This holistic approach addresses the complex needs of patients and promotes whole-person wellness.

2. Education and Training: Expanded education and training opportunities for healthcare professionals, including physicians, nurses, pharmacists, and naturopathic doctors, will increase awareness and competency in herbal medicine. Interprofessional collaboration and knowledge-sharing will enhance patient care and outcomes.

Sustainable Practices

1. Ethical Sourcing: Adoption of sustainable and ethical sourcing practices for medicinal herbs will promote biodiversity conservation, protect indigenous knowledge, and support local communities. Certification programs and traceability systems will ensure transparency and accountability throughout the supply chain.

2. Regenerative Agriculture: Emphasis on regenerative agriculture and agroecological principles will promote soil health, carbon sequestration, and ecosystem resilience. Agroforestry, permaculture, and organic farming methods will enhance the quality and potency of medicinal plants while mitigating environmental impact.

Technological Innovation

1. Herbal Analytics: Development of advanced analytical techniques, such as mass spectrometry, chromatography, and spectroscopy, will enable accurate identification, standardization, and quality control of herbal products. High-throughput screening methods will expedite the discovery of bioactive compounds and synergistic herbal combinations.

2. Digital Health Tools: Integration of digital health tools, such as mobile apps, wearable devices, and telemedicine platforms, will empower individuals to monitor their health, track herbal intake, and access personalized wellness recommendations. Artificial intelligence and machine learning algorithms will analyze big data to identify patterns and optimize treatment protocols.

Global Health Equity

1. Access to Herbal Medicine: Efforts to improve access to herbal medicine in underserved communities, both domestically and globally, will promote health equity and social justice. Affordable pricing, community-based clinics, and public health initiatives will expand access to herbal remedies and traditional healing modalities.

2. Cultural Competency: Cultural competency training and cross-cultural exchange programs will foster mutual respect, understanding, and collaboration among diverse healthcare practitioners and traditional healers. Culturally sensitive approaches to herbal medicine will honor indigenous wisdom and cultural traditions.

In conclusion, the future of herbal medicine holds tremendous promise for advancing healthcare, promoting sustainability, and fostering global health equity. Through evidence-based research, personalized medicine, integrative healthcare, sustainable practices, technological innovation, and a commitment to cultural competency, we can harness the full potential of herbal medicine to enhance human health and well-being while preserving the natural world for future generations. Let us embrace this journey with curiosity, collaboration, and a shared vision of a healthier, more harmonious world.

Glossary of Herbal Terms

1. Adaptogen: A natural substance that helps the body adapt to stress and maintain balance. Adaptogenic herbs, such as ashwagandha and rhodiola, support the body's resilience and promote overall well-being.

2. Decoction: A method of extracting medicinal compounds from herbs by simmering them in water over low heat for an extended period. Decoctions are commonly used for hard, woody, or fibrous herbs.

3. Infusion: A method of extracting medicinal compounds from herbs by steeping them in hot water for a short period. Infusions are typically used for delicate or aromatic herbs, such as flowers and leaves.

4. Tincture: A concentrated liquid extract of herbs, usually made by soaking herbs in alcohol or glycerin to extract their medicinal properties. Tinctures are convenient and shelf-stable and can be easily dosed.

5. Syrup: A sweet, viscous liquid made by combining herbal extracts or infusions with a sugar or honey base. Herbal syrups are commonly used to soothe coughs, sore throats, and respiratory congestion.

6. Salve: A semi-solid ointment or balm made by combining herbal-infused oils with beeswax or another thickening agent. Herbal salves are applied topically to soothe skin irritation, promote healing, and relieve discomfort.

7. Poultice: A soft, moist mass of herbs applied directly to the skin to alleviate pain, inflammation, or swelling. Poultices are typically made by mashing or blending fresh or dried herbs with water or another liquid.

8. Dried Herb: Herbs that have been harvested and dried for preservation. Drying herbs removes moisture and helps concentrate their flavor and medicinal properties for long-term storage and use.

9. Fresh Herb: Herbs that are harvested and used in their natural state, without drying or processing. Fresh herbs have a vibrant flavor and aroma and can be used in cooking, teas, and herbal preparations.

10. Botanical Name: The scientific name of a plant species, consisting of a genus and species epithet. Botanical names are standardized and provide a precise way to identify plants, regardless of

language or region.

11. Infusion Time: The length of time herbs are steeped in hot water to extract their medicinal properties. Infusion times vary depending on the type of herb and the desired strength of the infusion.

12. Dosage: The amount of herbal remedy or preparation recommended for therapeutic use. Dosage guidelines vary depending on factors such as age, weight, and health status.

13. Herbalism: The practice of using plants and plant-derived substances for medicinal purposes. Herbalism encompasses a wide range of traditions, from traditional folk remedies to modern scientific approaches.

14. Materia Medica: A comprehensive reference guide or database containing information about medicinal plants, including their properties, uses, preparations, and dosage recommendations.

15. Wildcrafting: The practice of sustainably harvesting medicinal plants from their natural habitats. Wildcrafters gather plants ethically, respecting local ecosystems and regulations to ensure the long-term viability of wild populations.

16. Standardization: The process of ensuring the consistency and potency of herbal products by controlling the levels of active compounds present. Standardization helps guarantee the quality and effectiveness of herbal remedies.

17. Synergistic: Refers to the combined effect of multiple herbs or compounds working together to produce a stronger or more beneficial outcome than any single component alone. Synergistic interactions enhance the overall efficacy of herbal preparations.

18. Contraindication: A specific situation or condition in which a particular herb or herbal remedy should not be used due to potential adverse effects or interactions. Contraindications may vary depending on individual health factors.

19. Side Effect: An unintended or unwanted effect of using an herbal remedy, which may occur in addition to its desired therapeutic effects. Side effects can range from mild to severe and may vary depending on individual sensitivity and dosage.

20. Toxicity: The degree to which a substance, including herbs, can cause harm or adverse effects when ingested, applied topically, or otherwise used. Understanding the toxicity of herbs is essential for ensuring their safe and responsible use.

21. Quality Control: Measures and procedures implemented to ensure the purity, potency, and safety of herbal products. Quality control protocols may include testing for contaminants, standardizing production processes, and adhering to regulatory standards.

This glossary provides a foundational understanding of key terms and concepts related to herbal medicine, serving as a valuable reference for both novice and experienced practitioners alike.

Herbal Remedy Quick Reference Guide

This quick reference guide provides an overview of common herbal remedies and their uses. Please note that this guide is for informational purposes only and does not constitute medical advice. Consult with a healthcare professional before using any herbal remedies, especially if you have preexisting health conditions or are taking medications.

Chamomile (Matricaria chamomilla)

- Uses: Promotes relaxation, relieves stress and anxiety, aids digestion, soothes upset stomach, supports sleep quality.
- Preparations: Herbal tea, tincture, essential oil, topical cream.

Echinacea (Echinacea purpurea)

- Uses: Boosts immune function, reduces the severity and duration of colds and flu, supports respiratory health.
- Preparations: Tincture, capsules, herbal tea.

Ginger (Zingiber officinale)

- Uses: Relieves nausea and motion sickness, aids digestion, reduces inflammation, supports circulation.
- Preparations: Fresh or dried root (tea, infusion), capsules, tincture.

Lavender (Lavandula angustifolia)

- Uses: Promotes relaxation and stress relief, relieves headaches, soothes skin irritation, supports sleep quality.
- Preparations: Essential oil (aromatherapy, topical use), herbal tea, tincture.

Peppermint (Mentha x piperita)

- Uses: Relieves digestive discomfort (gas, bloating, indigestion), eases tension headaches, supports respiratory health.
- Preparations: Herbal tea, essential oil (aromatherapy, topical use), capsules.

Valerian (Valeriana officinalis)

- Uses: Promotes relaxation and restful sleep, reduces anxiety and nervous tension, eases muscle tension and spasms.
- Preparations: Tincture, capsules, herbal tea.

Turmeric (Curcuma longa)

- Uses: Reduces inflammation and pain, supports joint health, aids digestion, boosts immune function.
- Preparations: Fresh or dried root (tea, infusion), capsules, powdered spice.

St. John's Wort (Hypericum perforatum)

- Uses: Alleviates symptoms of mild to moderate depression, reduces anxiety, supports mood balance.
- Preparations: Tincture, capsules, herbal tea (consult with healthcare provider due to potential interactions).

Lemon Balm (Melissa officinalis)

- Uses: Calms nerves and reduces anxiety, promotes relaxation and sleep, supports digestive health.
- Preparations: Herbal tea, tincture, essential oil (aromatherapy, topical use).

Garlic (Allium sativum)

- Uses: Supports cardiovascular health, boosts immune function, fights infection (antibacterial, antiviral), lowers blood pressure and cholesterol.
- Preparations: Fresh cloves (eaten raw or cooked), capsules, aged garlic extract.

Rosemary (Rosmarinus officinalis)

- Uses: Improves cognitive function and memory, supports mood balance, relieves muscle pain and tension.
- Preparations: Herbal tea, essential oil (aromatherapy, topical use), culinary seasoning.

Hawthorn (Crataegus spp.)

- Uses: Supports cardiovascular health, regulates blood pressure, strengthens the heart muscle, improves circulation.
- Preparations: Tincture, capsules, herbal tea.

Calendula (Calendula officinalis)

- Uses: Promotes wound healing and tissue repair, soothes skin inflammation and irritation, supports digestive health.
- Preparations: Herbal salve or cream, infused oil, herbal tea.

Nettle (Urtica dioica)

- Uses: Supports kidney and urinary tract health, reduces allergy symptoms, boosts energy and vitality.
- Preparations: Herbal tea, tincture, capsules, cooked greens (young leaves).

Dandelion (Taraxacum officinale)

- Uses: Supports liver and digestive health, aids detoxification, promotes fluid balance, boosts nutrient absorption.
- Preparations: Herbal tea (leaves and roots), tincture, capsules, culinary greens.

Passionflower (Passiflora incarnata)

- Uses: Calms nerves and reduces anxiety, promotes relaxation and sleep, eases muscle tension and spasms.
- Preparations: Tincture, capsules, herbal tea.

Licorice (Glycyrrhiza glabra)

- Uses: Soothes sore throat and cough, supports adrenal health, aids digestion, reduces inflammation.
- Preparations: Herbal tea, capsules, powdered root (used sparingly due to potential side effects).

Sage (Salvia officinalis)

- Uses: Relieves sore throat and cough, supports memory and cognitive function, promotes digestive health.
- Preparations: Herbal tea, culinary seasoning, essential oil (aromatherapy, topical use).

Marshmallow (Althaea officinalis)

- Uses: Soothes sore throat and cough, relieves digestive discomfort, supports urinary tract health.
- Preparations: Herbal tea, tincture, capsules.

Astragalus (Astragalus membranaceus)

- Uses: Boosts immune function, supports respiratory health, enhances energy and vitality.
- Preparations: Tincture, capsules, herbal tea.

This quick reference guide offers a glimpse into the diverse world of herbal remedies and their applications for promoting health and well-being. Experiment with different herbs and preparations to discover what works best for

Resources for Further Learning

Expanding your knowledge of herbal medicine can be an enriching journey filled with diverse perspectives, practical skills, and valuable insights. Whether you're a beginner or an experienced herbalist, these resources offer a wealth of information to deepen your understanding and proficiency in herbalism:

Books

1. "The Herbal Medicine-Maker's Handbook" by James Green: A comprehensive guide to making herbal preparations, including tinctures, salves, and teas, with detailed instructions and recipes.

2. "Rosemary Gladstar's Medicinal Herbs: A Beginner's Guide" by Rosemary Gladstar: An accessible introduction to herbalism, covering basic principles, common herbs, and practical applications for health and wellness.

3. "Adaptogens: Herbs for Strength, Stamina, and Stress Relief" by David Winston and Steven Maimes: A thorough exploration of adaptogenic herbs and their role in supporting resilience, vitality, and overall well-being.

4. "Medical Herbalism: The Science and Practice of Herbal Medicine" by David Hoffmann: A comprehensive textbook on herbal medicine, blending traditional wisdom with modern scientific research and clinical practice.

5. "The Modern Herbal Dispensatory: A Medicine-Making Guide" by Thomas Easley and Steven Horne: A practical handbook for creating herbal remedies at home, including step-by-step instructions, dosage guidelines, and safety precautions.

Online Courses

1. Herbal Academy: Offers online courses and programs for herbalists of all levels, covering topics such as materia medica, herbal formulation, wildcrafting, and clinical herbalism.

2. The School of Evolutionary Herbalism: Provides in-depth courses on holistic herbalism, plant energetics, constitutional assessment, and clinical skills, with a focus on traditional wisdom and evolutionary perspectives.

3. United Plant Savers: Offers educational resources, webinars, and workshops on plant conservation, ethical wildcrafting, and sustainable herbalism, with an emphasis on preserving native medicinal plants.

4. North American Institute of Medical Herbalism: Provides distance learning programs and clinical training in medical herbalism, including anatomy, physiology, pathology, and herbal therapeutics.

5. The Herbal Academy of New England: Offers online courses, workshops, and mentorship programs on herbalism, botany, wildcrafting, and herbal formulation, with a focus on hands-on learning and practical skills.

Podcasts

1. The Plant Path Podcast: Hosted by herbalist and educator Sajah Popham, this podcast explores the world of herbalism, plant medicine, and holistic health through interviews, discussions, and storytelling.

2. The Herbal Highway: Produced by KPFA Radio, this podcast features interviews with herbalists, botanists, and healers from diverse cultural backgrounds, sharing their wisdom and perspectives on herbal medicine.

3. HerbRally Podcast: Hosted by herbalist Mason Hutchison, this podcast covers a wide range of topics in herbalism, including plant identification, herbal traditions, ethical wildcrafting, and herbal business.

4. The Plant Medicine Podcast: Hosted by herbalist and educator Jesse Hardin, this podcast explores the therapeutic uses of medicinal plants, featuring interviews with herbalists, doctors, and researchers.

5. Real Herbalism Radio: Hosted by herbalists Sue Sierralupe and Candace Hunter, this podcast offers practical advice, tips, and insights on herbalism, gardening, and holistic health.

Websites and Online Resources

1. American Herbalists Guild (AHG): Provides educational resources, articles, and directories for herbalists, as well as information on professional standards and training programs.

2. Herbal Academy Blog: Offers a wealth of articles, recipes, and tutorials on herbalism, covering topics such as herbal remedies, plant identification, and herbal gardening.

3. Botanical Medicine Resources: Curated by herbalist and author Michael Moore, this website offers a collection of articles, monographs, and educational resources on medicinal plants and herbal medicine.

4. PubMed: A database of scientific research articles and studies on herbal medicine, providing valuable insights into the efficacy, safety, and mechanisms of action of medicinal plants.

5. YouTube Channels: Explore herbalism tutorials, plant identification guides, and educational videos on channels such as Herbal Jedi, Herbal Wisdom Institute, and The School of Evolutionary Herbalism.

These resources offer a diverse array of learning opportunities for herbalists and enthusiasts alike, providing valuable insights, practical skills, and inspiration for exploring the world of herbal medicine. Whether you prefer books, online courses, podcasts, or websites, there's something for everyone to deepen their understanding and appreciation of plant-based healing. Happy learning!

BONUS CONTENT:

Boosting testosterone levels naturally can support overall health and vitality. While herbal remedies can play a role in this process, it's essential to approach testosterone support holistically, incorporating lifestyle changes such as exercise, diet, and stress management. Here are some herbal remedies that may help boost testosterone levels:

1. Ashwagandha (Withania somnifera)
- Benefits: Known as an adaptogen, ashwagandha helps the body adapt to stress and may support healthy testosterone levels.
- How to Use: Take as a powdered root extract, tincture, or capsule. Follow dosage recommendations on the product label.

2. Tribulus Terrestris
- Benefits: Traditionally used to enhance libido and athletic performance, tribulus terrestris may also support testosterone levels.
- How to Use: Available as a supplement in various forms, including capsules, powders, and tinctures.

3. Fenugreek (Trigonella foenum-graecum)
- Benefits: Fenugreek seeds contain compounds that may help boost testosterone levels and improve libido.
- How to Use: Take as a supplement or incorporate fenugreek seeds into cooking or herbal teas.

4. Tongkat Ali (Eurycoma longifolia)
- Benefits: Also known as longjack, tongkat ali is believed to support testosterone production and improve sexual health.
- How to Use: Typically consumed as a powdered root extract or in capsule form.

5. Maca (Lepidium meyenii)
- Benefits: Maca root is known for its hormone-balancing properties and may help support healthy testosterone levels.
- How to Use: Add maca powder to smoothies, oatmeal, or beverages, or take it in capsule form.

6. Ginseng (Panax ginseng)
- Benefits: Ginseng may support testosterone production and improve energy levels and stamina.
- How to Use: Take as a standardized extract, tincture, or capsule.

7. Horny Goat Weed (Epimedium)
- Benefits: Traditionally used as an aphrodisiac, horny goat weed may help support testosterone levels and enhance sexual function.
- How to Use: Available in supplement form, including capsules and tinctures.

8. Pine Pollen
- Benefits: Pine pollen contains phytoandrogens, which are plant-based compounds that mimic testosterone in the body and may support hormonal balance.
- How to Use: Take as a powdered supplement or tincture.

9. Mucuna Pruriens
- Benefits: Mucuna pruriens contains L-dopa, a precursor to dopamine, which may help support healthy testosterone levels and improve mood.
- How to Use: Available in powdered form, capsules, or tinctures.

10. Saw Palmetto (Serenoa repens)
- Benefits: Saw palmetto may help support prostate health and balance hormone levels, including testosterone.
- How to Use: Typically taken as a standardized extract or in capsule form.

Important Considerations:
- Consult a Healthcare Professional: Before starting any herbal supplement regimen, especially for hormonal support, consult with a healthcare professional to ensure it's safe and appropriate for you.
- Quality and Dosage: Choose high-quality supplements from reputable brands and follow dosage recommendations carefully.
- Holistic Approach: Herbal remedies work best when combined with lifestyle changes such as regular exercise, a balanced diet, stress management, and adequate sleep.

By incorporating these herbal remedies into a holistic approach to health and wellness, you can support healthy testosterone levels and overall vitality.

Managing symptoms of menopause with herbal remedies can provide relief for many women. However, it's crucial to consult with a healthcare professional before starting any herbal regimen, especially if you have underlying health conditions or are taking medications. Here are some herbal remedies commonly used to alleviate symptoms of menopause:

1. Black Cohosh (Actaea racemosa)
- Benefits: Black cohosh is often used to relieve hot flashes, night sweats, and mood swings associated with menopause.
- How to Use: Available in various forms, including capsules, tablets, tinctures, and teas. Follow dosage recommendations on the product label.

2. Red Clover (Trifolium pratense)
- Benefits: Red clover contains compounds called isoflavones, which may help reduce hot flashes and improve bone health during menopause.
- How to Use: Enjoy as a tea or take as a standardized extract or capsule.

3. Dong Quai (Angelica sinensis)
- Benefits: Dong quai is commonly used in traditional Chinese medicine to relieve symptoms of menopause, including hot flashes, vaginal dryness, and mood swings.
- How to Use: Available as a tincture, capsule, or dried root for tea.

4. Evening Primrose Oil (Oenothera biennis)
- Benefits: Evening primrose oil contains gamma-linolenic acid (GLA), which may help alleviate symptoms of menopause such as hot flashes and breast tenderness.
- How to Use: Take as a supplement in softgel form. Follow dosage recommendations on the product label.

5. Sage (Salvia officinalis)
- Benefits: Sage has a long history of use in herbal medicine for reducing hot flashes and night sweats associated with menopause.
- How to Use: Enjoy as a tea or use as a culinary herb. Sage supplements are also available in capsule form.

6. Chasteberry (Vitex agnus-castus)
- Benefits: Chasteberry may help regulate hormone levels and alleviate symptoms such as hot flashes, mood swings, and irregular periods during menopause.
- How to Use: Take as a tincture or in capsule form.

7. Ginseng (Panax ginseng)
- Benefits: Ginseng may help improve energy levels, mood, and cognitive function during menopause.
- How to Use: Take as a standardized extract or in capsule form.

8. St. John's Wort (Hypericum perforatum)
- Benefits: St. John's wort may help alleviate mood swings, anxiety, and depression commonly experienced during menopause.
- How to Use: Take as a standardized extract or in capsule form.

9. Licorice Root (Glycyrrhiza glabra)
- Benefits: Licorice root may help support hormone balance and alleviate symptoms such as hot flashes and mood swings.
- How to Use: Enjoy as a tea or take as a tincture. Follow dosage recommendations on the product label.

10. Motherwort (Leonurus cardiaca)
- Benefits: Motherwort is traditionally used to relieve symptoms of menopause, including hot flashes, anxiety, and insomnia.
- How to Use: Take as a tincture or in capsule form.

Important Considerations:
- Consult with a Healthcare Professional: Before starting any herbal remedy regimen for menopause, consult with a healthcare professional to ensure it's safe and appropriate for you, especially if you have underlying health conditions or are taking medications.
- Quality and Dosage: Choose high-quality supplements from reputable brands and follow dosage recommendations carefully.
    - Holistic Approach: Herbal remedies work best when combined with lifestyle changes such as regular exercise, a balanced diet, stress management, and adequate sleep.
    -

Herbal remedies can be a supportive addition to a healthy lifestyle for weight loss. However, it's essential to approach weight loss holistically, incorporating a balanced diet, regular exercise, adequate sleep, and stress management. Here are some herbal remedies that may aid in weight loss:

1. Green Tea (Camellia sinensis)
- Benefits: Green tea contains catechins and caffeine, which may boost metabolism and increase fat burning.
- How to Use: Enjoy as a hot or cold beverage, or take as a standardized extract or supplement.

2. Garcinia Cambogia (Garcinia gummi-gutta)

- Benefits: Garcinia cambogia contains hydroxycitric acid (HCA), which may suppress appetite and inhibit fat storage.
- How to Use: Take as a standardized extract or supplement. Follow dosage recommendations on the product label.

3. Cinnamon (Cinnamomum verum)
- Benefits: Cinnamon may help regulate blood sugar levels and reduce cravings for sweet foods, potentially aiding in weight management.
- How to Use: Add cinnamon powder to foods and beverages, or take as a supplement.

4. Cayenne Pepper (Capsicum annuum)
- Benefits: Cayenne pepper contains capsaicin, which may increase metabolism and promote fat burning.
- How to Use: Add cayenne pepper to meals and recipes, or take as a supplement.

5. Ginger (Zingiber officinale)
- Benefits: Ginger has thermogenic properties that may increase calorie burning and reduce appetite.
- How to Use: Enjoy fresh ginger in teas, smoothies, and dishes, or take as a supplement.

6. Dandelion (Taraxacum officinale)
- Benefits: Dandelion may support weight loss by acting as a diuretic and promoting detoxification.
- How to Use: Enjoy dandelion tea or add fresh dandelion leaves to salads and meals.

7. Gymnema Sylvestre
- Benefits: Gymnema sylvestre may help reduce sugar cravings and support balanced blood sugar levels, aiding in weight management.
- How to Use: Take as a standardized extract or supplement.

8. Fenugreek (Trigonella foenum-graecum)
- Benefits: Fenugreek seeds contain soluble fiber, which may promote feelings of fullness and reduce calorie intake.
- How to Use: Add fenugreek seeds to meals, or take as a supplement.

9. Guggul (Commiphora mukul)
- Benefits: Guggul extract may help support thyroid function and metabolism, potentially aiding in weight loss.
- How to Use: Take as a standardized extract or supplement.

10. Lemon Balm (Melissa officinalis)
- Benefits: Lemon balm may help reduce stress and emotional eating, supporting weight management efforts.
- How to Use: Enjoy lemon balm tea or take as a supplement.

Important Considerations:
- Consult with a Healthcare Professional: Before starting any herbal remedy regimen for weight loss, consult with a healthcare professional to ensure it's safe and appropriate for you, especially if you have underlying health conditions or are taking medications.
- Quality and Dosage: Choose high-quality supplements from reputable brands and follow dosage recommendations carefully.
- Healthy Lifestyle: Herbal remedies work best when combined with a balanced diet, regular exercise, adequate sleep, and stress management practices.

Erectile dysfunction (ED) can have various underlying causes, including physical, psychological, and lifestyle factors. While herbal remedies may help improve blood flow, hormone balance, and overall sexual function, it's essential to address any underlying health issues and consult with a healthcare professional before starting any herbal regimen. Here are some herbal remedies that may support better erections:

1. Panax Ginseng (Asian Ginseng)
- Benefits: Panax ginseng may improve erectile function by promoting nitric oxide production, which relaxes blood vessels and increases blood flow to the penis.
- How to Use: Take as a standardized extract or supplement. Follow dosage recommendations on the product label.

2. Horny Goat Weed (Epimedium)
- Benefits: Horny goat weed contains icariin, a compound that may help improve blood flow to the penis and enhance sexual function.
- How to Use: Take as a standardized extract or supplement. Follow dosage recommendations on the product label.

3. L-arginine
- Benefits: L-arginine is an amino acid that the body converts into nitric oxide, which helps dilate blood vessels and improve blood flow, potentially leading to better erections.
- How to Use: Take as a supplement. Follow dosage recommendations on the product label.

4. Tribulus Terrestris
- Benefits: Tribulus terrestris may help increase testosterone levels and improve libido and sexual function in men with ED.
- How to Use: Take as a standardized extract or supplement. Follow dosage recommendations on the product label.

5. Yohimbe Bark (Pausinystalia yohimbe)
- Benefits: Yohimbe bark contains yohimbine, a compound that may improve erectile function by increasing blood flow to the penis and enhancing sexual arousal.
- How to Use: Take as a standardized extract or supplement. Use caution and follow dosage recommendations carefully, as yohimbe can have side effects and interactions with medications.

6. Maca (Lepidium meyenii)
- Benefits: Maca root may help improve sexual function and libido by balancing hormone levels and increasing energy and stamina.
- How to Use: Take as a powdered root extract or supplement. Follow dosage recommendations on the product label.

7. Ginkgo Biloba
- Benefits: Ginkgo biloba may improve blood circulation and increase blood flow to the penis, potentially enhancing erectile function.
- How to Use: Take as a standardized extract or supplement. Follow dosage recommendations on the product label.

8. Ashwagandha (Withania somnifera)
- Benefits: Ashwagandha is an adaptogenic herb that may help reduce stress and anxiety, which can contribute to erectile dysfunction.
- How to Use: Take as a standardized extract or supplement. Follow dosage recommendations on the product label.

Important Considerations:
- Consult with a Healthcare Professional: Before starting any herbal remedy regimen for erectile dysfunction, consult with a healthcare professional to ensure it's safe and appropriate for you, especially if you have underlying health conditions or are taking medications.
- Quality and Dosage: Choose high-quality supplements from reputable brands and follow dosage recommendations carefully.
- Lifestyle Factors: Addressing lifestyle factors such as diet, exercise, stress management, and sleep quality can also play a significant role in improving erectile function.

Herbal remedies can be effective in alleviating headaches, especially when the cause is tension, stress, or mild inflammation. However, it's essential to determine the underlying cause of your headaches and consult with a healthcare professional if you experience severe or chronic headaches. Here are some herbal remedies that may help relieve headaches:

1. Feverfew (Tanacetum parthenium)
- Benefits: Feverfew contains compounds that may help reduce inflammation and prevent migraines.
- How to Use: Take as a standardized extract or supplement. Follow dosage recommendations on the product label.

2. Peppermint (Mentha x piperita)
- Benefits: Peppermint has a cooling effect and contains menthol, which can help relax muscles and relieve tension headaches.
- How to Use: Drink peppermint tea or inhale peppermint essential oil for aromatherapy. You can also apply diluted peppermint oil to the temples for topical relief.

3. Ginger (Zingiber officinale)
- Benefits: Ginger has anti-inflammatory properties and may help reduce migraine symptoms and relieve nausea associated with headaches.
- How to Use: Drink ginger tea, chew on a piece of fresh ginger, or take ginger supplements. You can also apply ginger essential oil to the temples for topical relief.

4. Willow Bark (Salix spp.)
- Benefits: Willow bark contains salicin, a compound similar to aspirin, which may help reduce pain and inflammation associated with headaches.
- How to Use: Take as a standardized extract or supplement. Follow dosage recommendations on the product label.

5. Lavender (Lavandula angustifolia)
- Benefits: Lavender has calming and sedative properties that may help reduce stress and tension headaches.
- How to Use: Inhale lavender essential oil for aromatherapy, add a few drops to a warm bath, or apply diluted lavender oil to the temples for topical relief.

6. Butterbur (Petasites hybridus)
- Benefits: Butterbur contains compounds called petasins, which may help reduce the frequency and severity of migraines.
- How to Use: Take as a standardized extract or supplement. Follow dosage recommendations on the product label.

7. Chamomile (Matricaria chamomilla)

- Benefits: Chamomile has anti-inflammatory and calming properties that may help reduce tension and stress headaches.
- How to Use: Drink chamomile tea or inhale chamomile essential oil for aromatherapy. You can also apply diluted chamomile oil to the temples for topical relief.

8. Valerian (Valeriana officinalis)
- Benefits: Valerian has muscle-relaxing and sedative properties that may help alleviate tension headaches and promote relaxation.
- How to Use: Drink valerian tea or take valerian supplements. Follow dosage recommendations on the product label.

9. Lemon Balm (Melissa officinalis)
- Benefits: Lemon balm has calming and anti-inflammatory properties that may help relieve headaches caused by stress or tension.
- How to Use: Drink lemon balm tea or inhale lemon balm essential oil for aromatherapy. You can also apply diluted lemon balm oil to the temples for topical relief.

Important Considerations:
- Consult with a Healthcare Professional: If you experience severe or chronic headaches, consult with a healthcare professional to determine the underlying cause and appropriate treatment plan.
- Safety Precautions: Some herbs may interact with medications or have side effects, so it's
Herbal remedies can help alleviate symptoms and support the immune system during a cold. While they may not cure the cold virus, they can provide relief from symptoms such as congestion, sore throat, and cough. Here are some herbal remedies that may help:

1. Echinacea (Echinacea purpurea)
- Benefits: Echinacea is believed to stimulate the immune system and reduce the severity and duration of cold symptoms.
- How to Use: Take echinacea supplements or drink echinacea tea. Follow dosage recommendations on the product label.

2. Elderberry (Sambucus nigra)
- Benefits: Elderberry is rich in antioxidants and may help reduce inflammation and relieve cold symptoms, including congestion and cough.
- How to Use: Take elderberry syrup or supplements. Follow dosage recommendations on the product label.

3. Ginger (Zingiber officinale)
- Benefits: Ginger has anti-inflammatory and antimicrobial properties that may help soothe sore throat, reduce cough, and alleviate nausea associated with colds.
- How to Use: Drink ginger tea or add fresh ginger to soups and meals.

4. Garlic (Allium sativum)
- Benefits: Garlic has antimicrobial properties and may help boost the immune system and reduce the severity of cold symptoms.
- How to Use: Consume raw garlic cloves or add garlic to your meals for added flavor and health benefits.

5. Honey
- Benefits: Honey has antimicrobial and soothing properties that may help relieve sore throat and cough associated with colds.
- How to Use: Add honey to hot tea or warm water with lemon. Do not give honey to children under

one year of age.

6. Peppermint (Mentha x piperita)
- Benefits: Peppermint has decongestant properties that may help relieve nasal congestion and sinus pressure associated with colds.
- How to Use: Drink peppermint tea or inhale peppermint essential oil for aromatherapy.

7. Chamomile (Matricaria chamomilla)
- Benefits: Chamomile has anti-inflammatory and soothing properties that may help relieve sore throat and promote relaxation during illness.
- How to Use: Drink chamomile tea or inhale chamomile essential oil for aromatherapy.

8. Thyme (Thymus vulgaris)
- Benefits: Thyme has antimicrobial properties and may help relieve cough and congestion associated with colds.
- How to Use: Drink thyme tea or inhale thyme essential oil for aromatherapy.

9. Licorice Root (Glycyrrhiza glabra)
- Benefits: Licorice root has soothing properties that may help relieve sore throat and cough associated with colds.
- How to Use: Drink licorice root tea or chew on licorice root sticks.

10. Oregano (Origanum vulgare)
- Benefits: Oregano contains compounds with antimicrobial properties that may help fight off cold viruses and reduce the severity of symptoms.
- How to Use: Drink oregano tea or add fresh oregano to your meals for added flavor and health benefits.

Important Considerations:
- Consult with a Healthcare Professional: If you have a severe or persistent cold, or if you have underlying health conditions, consult with a healthcare professional before using herbal remedies.
- Hydration and Rest: In addition to herbal remedies, make sure to stay hydrated, get plenty of rest, and practice good hygiene to support recovery from a cold.

Herbal remedies can provide relief from symptoms and support the immune system during the flu. While they may not cure the flu virus, they can help alleviate symptoms such as fever, cough, congestion, and fatigue. Here are some herbal remedies that may help:

1. Echinacea (Echinacea purpurea)
- Benefits: Echinacea is believed to stimulate the immune system and reduce the severity and duration of flu symptoms.
- How to Use: Take echinacea supplements or drink echinacea tea. Follow dosage recommendations on the product label.

2. Elderberry (Sambucus nigra)
- Benefits: Elderberry is rich in antioxidants and may help reduce inflammation and relieve flu symptoms, including fever, cough, and congestion.
- How to Use: Take elderberry syrup or supplements. Follow dosage recommendations on the product label.

3. Ginger (Zingiber officinale)
- Benefits: Ginger has anti-inflammatory and antimicrobial properties that may help soothe sore

throat, reduce cough, and alleviate nausea associated with the flu.
- How to Use: Drink ginger tea or add fresh ginger to soups and meals.

4. Garlic (Allium sativum)
- Benefits: Garlic has antimicrobial properties and may help boost the immune system and reduce the severity of flu symptoms.
- How to Use: Consume raw garlic cloves or add garlic to your meals for added flavor and health benefits.

5. Honey
- Benefits: Honey has antimicrobial and soothing properties that may help relieve sore throat and cough associated with the flu.
- How to Use: Add honey to hot tea or warm water with lemon. Do not give honey to children under one year of age.

6. Peppermint (Mentha x piperita)
- Benefits: Peppermint has decongestant properties that may help relieve nasal congestion and sinus pressure associated with the flu.
- How to Use: Drink peppermint tea or inhale peppermint essential oil for aromatherapy.

7. Chamomile (Matricaria chamomilla)
- Benefits: Chamomile has anti-inflammatory and soothing properties that may help relieve sore throat and promote relaxation during illness.
- How to Use: Drink chamomile tea or inhale chamomile essential oil for aromatherapy.

8. Thyme (Thymus vulgaris)
- Benefits: Thyme has antimicrobial properties and may help relieve cough and congestion associated with the flu.
- How to Use: Drink thyme tea or inhale thyme essential oil for aromatherapy.

9. Licorice Root (Glycyrrhiza glabra)
- Benefits: Licorice root has soothing properties that may help relieve sore throat and cough associated with the flu.
- How to Use: Drink licorice root tea or chew on licorice root sticks.

10. Oregano (Origanum vulgare)
- Benefits: Oregano contains compounds with antimicrobial properties that may help fight off flu viruses and reduce the severity of symptoms.
- How to Use: Drink oregano tea or add fresh oregano to your meals for added flavor and health benefits.

Important Considerations:
- Consult with a Healthcare Professional: If you have a severe case of the flu, or if you have underlying health conditions, consult with a healthcare professional before using herbal remedies.
- Hydration and Rest: In addition to herbal remedies, make sure to stay hydrated, get plenty of rest, and practice good hygiene to support recovery from the flu. If symptoms persist or worsen, seek medical attention promptly.

Herpes is a viral infection caused by the herpes simplex virus (HSV). While there's no cure for herpes, some herbal remedies may help alleviate symptoms and support the immune system. However, it's essential to consult with a healthcare professional before using herbal remedies, especially if you're managing a herpes outbreak. Here are some herbal remedies that may offer relief:

1. Lemon Balm (Melissa officinalis)
- Benefits: Lemon balm has antiviral properties and may help reduce the severity and duration of herpes outbreaks.
- How to Use: Apply lemon balm cream or ointment topically to affected areas during outbreaks. Drink lemon balm tea for added immune support.

2. Echinacea (Echinacea purpurea)
- Benefits: Echinacea is believed to stimulate the immune system and may help reduce the frequency and severity of herpes outbreaks.
- How to Use: Take echinacea supplements or drink echinacea tea regularly to support immune function.

3. Tea Tree Oil (Melaleuca alternifolia)
- Benefits: Tea tree oil has antiviral and anti-inflammatory properties that may help soothe herpes sores and promote healing.
- How to Use: Dilute tea tree oil with a carrier oil (such as coconut oil) and apply it topically to affected areas. Use with caution, as undiluted tea tree oil may irritate the skin.

4. Aloe Vera
- Benefits: Aloe vera has soothing and anti-inflammatory properties that may help relieve discomfort associated with herpes sores.
- How to Use: Apply aloe vera gel topically to affected areas for cooling relief. Use pure aloe vera gel or products containing a high concentration of aloe vera.

5. Licorice Root (Glycyrrhiza glabra)
- Benefits: Licorice root contains compounds that have antiviral and anti-inflammatory properties, which may help reduce herpes symptoms.
- How to Use: Apply licorice root cream or ointment topically to affected areas. Drink licorice root tea for added immune support.

6. Olive Leaf Extract (Olea europaea)
- Benefits: Olive leaf extract contains oleuropein, a compound with antiviral properties that may help inhibit the replication of the herpes virus.
- How to Use: Take olive leaf extract supplements according to the recommended dosage on the product label.

7. Peppermint Oil (Mentha x piperita)
- Benefits: Peppermint oil has cooling and antiviral properties that may help soothe herpes sores and reduce itching.
- How to Use: Dilute peppermint oil with a carrier oil and apply it topically to affected areas. Use with caution, as undiluted peppermint oil may irritate the skin.

Important Considerations:
- Consult with a Healthcare Professional: Herbal remedies may interact with medications or exacerbate certain health conditions. It's essential to consult with a healthcare professional before using herbal remedies, especially if you're managing a herpes outbreak or have underlying health concerns.
- Hygiene and Prevention: Practice good hygiene, including washing your hands frequently and avoiding touching herpes sores. Additionally, consider lifestyle changes and stress management techniques to help reduce the frequency and severity of herpes outbreaks.

- Avoid Triggers: Identify and avoid triggers that may exacerbate herpes outbreaks, such as stress, fatigue, and exposure to sunlight.

Hair loss can be distressing, and while herbal remedies may help support hair health and stimulate growth, it's essential to address any underlying causes and consult with a healthcare professional for proper diagnosis and treatment. Here are some herbal remedies that may help with hair loss:

1. Saw Palmetto (Serenoa repens)
- Benefits: Saw palmetto may help inhibit the conversion of testosterone to dihydrotestosterone (DHT), a hormone associated with hair loss, particularly in male and female pattern baldness.
- How to Use: Take saw palmetto supplements or use saw palmetto oil topically on the scalp. Follow dosage recommendations on the product label.

2. Rosemary (Rosmarinus officinalis)
- Benefits: Rosemary has been traditionally used to stimulate hair growth and improve scalp health. It contains compounds that may increase circulation to the scalp and promote hair follicle activity.
- How to Use: Make a rosemary-infused oil by steeping rosemary leaves in a carrier oil (such as olive or coconut oil) and applying it to the scalp. You can also use rosemary essential oil diluted in a carrier oil as a scalp massage oil.

3. Peppermint (Mentha x piperita)
- Benefits: Peppermint essential oil has cooling and stimulating properties that may help improve scalp circulation and promote hair growth.
- How to Use: Dilute peppermint essential oil in a carrier oil and massage it into the scalp. Leave it on for a few minutes before rinsing off. Use with caution, as peppermint oil may cause a tingling sensation.

4. Aloe Vera
- Benefits: Aloe vera has moisturizing and soothing properties that may help soothe the scalp, reduce inflammation, and promote healthy hair growth.
- How to Use: Apply pure aloe vera gel directly to the scalp and hair, leave it on for 30 minutes to an hour, then rinse off. You can also use aloe vera juice as a scalp rinse after shampooing.

5. Ginseng (Panax ginseng)
- Benefits: Ginseng has been used traditionally to promote hair growth and improve hair strength and texture. It contains compounds that may stimulate hair follicles and increase circulation to the scalp.
- How to Use: Take ginseng supplements or use ginseng extract topically on the scalp. Follow dosage recommendations on the product label.

6. Lavender (Lavandula angustifolia)
- Benefits: Lavender essential oil has antimicrobial and calming properties that may help improve scalp health and promote hair growth.
- How to Use: Dilute lavender essential oil in a carrier oil and massage it into the scalp. Leave it on overnight or for at least 30 minutes before rinsing off.

Important Considerations:
- Consult with a Healthcare Professional: Before using herbal remedies for hair loss, especially if you're experiencing significant or sudden hair loss, consult with a healthcare professional to rule out underlying medical conditions and determine the most appropriate treatment plan.
- Consistency is Key: Herbal remedies may take time to show results, so be patient and consistent with your chosen treatments. It may take several weeks or months to see noticeable improvements

in hair growth and scalp health.
- Holistic Approach: In addition to herbal remedies, maintain a healthy lifestyle with a balanced diet, regular exercise, adequate sleep, and stress management techniques to support overall hair health and well-being.

Herbal remedies can be a gentle and effective way to manage acne by addressing inflammation, killing bacteria, and balancing oil production. However, it's essential to test any new treatment on a small patch of skin and consult with a dermatologist before starting a new regimen, especially if you have sensitive skin or severe acne. Here are some herbal remedies that may help with acne:

1. Tea Tree Oil (Melaleuca alternifolia)
- Benefits: Tea tree oil has antimicrobial and anti-inflammatory properties that can help reduce acne-causing bacteria and inflammation.
- How to Use: Dilute tea tree oil with a carrier oil (such as coconut oil) and apply it directly to acne-prone areas using a cotton swab. Start with a small amount and increase if tolerated. Avoid applying near the eyes.

2. Witch Hazel (Hamamelis virginiana)
- Benefits: Witch hazel has astringent properties that can help tighten pores, reduce inflammation, and remove excess oil from the skin.
- How to Use: Apply witch hazel to the skin using a cotton ball or pad after cleansing. Use alcohol-free witch hazel to prevent drying out the skin.

3. Aloe Vera
- Benefits: Aloe vera has anti-inflammatory and soothing properties that can help calm redness and irritation associated with acne.
- How to Use: Apply pure aloe vera gel directly to acne-prone areas or use products containing aloe vera as an ingredient. Leave it on for 10-15 minutes before rinsing off with water.

4. Lavender (Lavandula angustifolia)
- Benefits: Lavender essential oil has antibacterial and anti-inflammatory properties that can help reduce acne and promote healing.
- How to Use: Dilute lavender essential oil with a carrier oil and apply it to acne-prone areas. Alternatively, add a few drops of lavender oil to a bowl of steaming water and use it for facial steaming.

5. Green Tea
- Benefits: Green tea contains antioxidants and anti-inflammatory compounds that can help reduce acne and soothe the skin.
- How to Use: Brew a cup of green tea and let it cool. Use a cotton ball to apply the tea to acne-prone areas or use green tea as a toner after cleansing.

6. Calendula (Calendula officinalis)
- Benefits: Calendula has anti-inflammatory and antimicrobial properties that can help soothe irritated skin and reduce acne.
- How to Use: Apply calendula cream or ointment to acne-prone areas. You can also make a calendula-infused oil by steeping dried calendula flowers in a carrier oil and applying it to the skin.

7. Neem (Azadirachta indica)
- Benefits: Neem has antibacterial, antifungal, and anti-inflammatory properties that can help treat acne and prevent breakouts.
- How to Use: Apply neem oil directly to acne-prone areas or use skincare products containing

neem extract. You can also make a neem face mask by mixing neem powder with water or honey.

Important Considerations:
- Patch Test: Before using any herbal remedy on your face, perform a patch test on a small area of skin to check for any allergic reactions or irritation.
- Consistency: Herbal remedies may take time to show results, so be patient and consistent with your chosen treatments. It may take several weeks or even months to see significant improvements in acne.
- Holistic Approach: In addition to herbal remedies, maintain a healthy skincare routine with gentle cleansing, exfoliation, and moisturizing. Avoid touching your face, and try to manage stress levels, as stress can exacerbate acne.

Herbal remedies can be a gentle and natural way to improve skin health by providing nourishment, hydration, and protection from environmental stressors. Incorporating herbs into your skincare routine can help address various skin concerns, such as dryness, inflammation, acne, and aging. Here are some herbal remedies that may promote better skin:

1. Chamomile (Matricaria chamomilla)
- Benefits: Chamomile has anti-inflammatory and soothing properties that can help calm irritated skin, reduce redness, and promote healing.
- How to Use: Brew chamomile tea and use it as a facial toner or mix chamomile essential oil with a carrier oil for a calming facial massage.

2. Calendula (Calendula officinalis)
- Benefits: Calendula has antibacterial, antifungal, and anti-inflammatory properties that can help soothe and heal various skin conditions, including acne, eczema, and minor wounds.
- How to Use: Apply calendula-infused oil or cream to the skin to promote healing and reduce inflammation.

3. Lavender (Lavandula angustifolia)
- Benefits: Lavender essential oil has antibacterial, antifungal, and anti-inflammatory properties that can help soothe irritated skin, reduce acne, and promote relaxation.
- How to Use: Dilute lavender essential oil with a carrier oil and apply it to the skin, or add a few drops to a warm bath for a calming soak.

4. Rosehip Seed Oil (Rosa canina)
- Benefits: Rosehip seed oil is rich in vitamins A, C, and E, as well as essential fatty acids, which can help hydrate the skin, improve elasticity, and reduce the appearance of scars and wrinkles.
- How to Use: Apply a few drops of rosehip seed oil to the skin after cleansing and toning, or mix it with your moisturizer for added hydration.

5. Green Tea
- Benefits: Green tea contains antioxidants and anti-inflammatory compounds that can help protect the skin from environmental damage, reduce inflammation, and promote collagen production.
- How to Use: Brew green tea and use it as a facial toner, or apply green tea extract topically to the skin for added antioxidant protection.

6. Witch Hazel (Hamamelis virginiana)
- Benefits: Witch hazel has astringent and anti-inflammatory properties that can help tighten pores, reduce inflammation, and soothe irritated skin.
- How to Use: Apply witch hazel to the skin using a cotton ball or pad after cleansing to remove excess oil and impurities.

7. Turmeric (Curcuma longa)
- Benefits: Turmeric contains curcumin, a compound with antioxidant and anti-inflammatory properties that can help brighten the skin, reduce acne, and promote healing.
- How to Use: Mix turmeric powder with honey or yogurt to create a nourishing face mask, or add a pinch of turmeric to your moisturizer for added benefits.

Important Considerations:
- Patch Test: Before using any herbal remedy on your face, perform a patch test on a small area of skin to check for any allergic reactions or irritation.
- Consistency: Consistent use of herbal remedies is key to seeing results. Incorporate them into your skincare routine and use them regularly for best results.
- Hydration and Sun Protection: Drink plenty of water to keep your skin hydrated from the inside out, and always wear sunscreen to protect your skin from sun damage.

Certainly! Here are some herbal remedies that may help alleviate constipation:

1. Aloe Vera
- Benefits: Aloe vera contains compounds that can help stimulate bowel movements and promote regularity.
- How to Use: Drink aloe vera juice according to the recommended dosage on the product label. Ensure that the product is intended for internal use and free from aloin, a laxative compound found in the outer leaf.

2. Senna (Cassia angustifolia)
- Benefits: Senna is a natural laxative herb that can help stimulate bowel movements and relieve constipation.
- How to Use: Take senna supplements or drink senna tea. Follow dosage recommendations carefully, as excessive use may lead to dependency.

3. Dandelion (Taraxacum officinale)
- Benefits: Dandelion root contains compounds that can help stimulate bile production and promote digestion, which may relieve constipation.
- How to Use: Drink dandelion root tea or take dandelion root supplements. You can also incorporate fresh dandelion leaves into salads.

4. Slippery Elm (Ulmus rubra)
- Benefits: Slippery elm contains mucilage, a gel-like substance that can help soften stool and promote bowel movements.
- How to Use: Take slippery elm supplements or mix slippery elm powder with water to make a soothing drink.

5. Psyllium Husk (Plantago ovata)
- Benefits: Psyllium husk is a soluble fiber that can help bulk up stool and promote regular bowel movements.
- How to Use: Mix psyllium husk powder with water and drink it immediately. Follow with another glass of water to ensure proper hydration.

6. Ginger (Zingiber officinale)
- Benefits: Ginger contains compounds that can help stimulate digestion and relieve gastrointestinal discomfort, including constipation.
- How to Use: Drink ginger tea or add fresh ginger to your meals for added flavor and health

benefits.

7. Fennel (Foeniculum vulgare)
- Benefits: Fennel seeds contain compounds that can help relax the muscles in the digestive tract and relieve gas and bloating, which may alleviate constipation.
- How to Use: Chew on fennel seeds after meals or drink fennel seed tea.

Important Considerations:
- Hydration: Drink plenty of water throughout the day to help soften stool and promote bowel movements.
- Fiber-Rich Diet: Eat a diet rich in fiber from fruits, vegetables, whole grains, and legumes to help bulk up stool and support regularity.
- Physical Activity: Engage in regular physical activity to help stimulate bowel movements and support overall digestive health.
- Consultation: Consult with a healthcare professional before using herbal remedies for constipation, especially if you have underlying health conditions or are taking medications. They can provide personalized recommendations based on your individual needs and medical history.

Herbal remedies can help alleviate symptoms of acid reflux by soothing the digestive tract, reducing inflammation, and promoting proper digestion. Here are some herbal remedies that may help:

1. Marshmallow Root (Althaea officinalis)
- Benefits: Marshmallow root contains mucilage, a gel-like substance that coats the lining of the esophagus and stomach, providing relief from heartburn and irritation.
- How to Use: Drink marshmallow root tea or take marshmallow root supplements. Allow the tea to cool slightly before drinking to maximize its soothing effects.

2. Slippery Elm (Ulmus rubra)
- Benefits: Slippery elm contains mucilage, which coats and soothes the digestive tract, reducing irritation and inflammation associated with acid reflux.
- How to Use: Take slippery elm supplements or mix slippery elm powder with water to create a soothing drink.

3. Ginger (Zingiber officinale)
- Benefits: Ginger has anti-inflammatory properties and can help reduce stomach acid production, alleviate nausea, and promote digestion.
- How to Use: Drink ginger tea, chew on fresh ginger slices, or take ginger supplements. Ginger can also be added to meals for flavor and digestive support.

4. Chamomile (Matricaria chamomilla)
- Benefits: Chamomile has anti-inflammatory and calming properties that can help reduce acid reflux symptoms and promote relaxation.
- How to Use: Drink chamomile tea before or after meals to soothe the digestive tract and reduce inflammation.

5. Licorice Root (Glycyrrhiza glabra)
- Benefits: Licorice root contains compounds that help protect the lining of the esophagus and stomach, reducing irritation and inflammation associated with acid reflux.
- How to Use: Drink licorice root tea or take licorice root supplements. Note that deglycyrrhizinated licorice (DGL) is often recommended to avoid potential side effects associated with regular licorice root.

6. Peppermint (Mentha x piperita)
- Benefits: Peppermint has a calming effect on the digestive tract and can help relieve symptoms of acid reflux, including indigestion and bloating.
- How to Use: Drink peppermint tea or chew on fresh peppermint leaves. However, avoid peppermint if you have gastroesophageal reflux disease (GERD), as it can relax the lower esophageal sphincter and worsen symptoms.

Important Considerations:
- Diet and Lifestyle: In addition to herbal remedies, maintain a healthy diet and lifestyle to manage acid reflux. Avoid trigger foods such as spicy, acidic, and fatty foods, and limit caffeine and alcohol intake. Eat smaller, more frequent meals, and avoid lying down immediately after eating.
- Consultation: Consult with a healthcare professional before using herbal remedies for acid reflux, especially if you have underlying health conditions or are taking medications. They can provide personalized recommendations based on your individual needs and medical history.

Herbal remedies can help alleviate congestion by promoting sinus drainage, reducing inflammation, and providing relief from nasal congestion and sinus pressure. Here are some herbal remedies that may help:

1. Eucalyptus (Eucalyptus globulus)
- Benefits: Eucalyptus contains cineole, a compound that can help thin mucus, reduce inflammation, and provide relief from nasal congestion.
- How to Use: Add a few drops of eucalyptus essential oil to a bowl of hot water and inhale the steam. You can also diffuse eucalyptus essential oil in the air or use eucalyptus-based chest rubs.

2. Peppermint (Mentha x piperita)
- Benefits: Peppermint has menthol, which can help open up the nasal passages, relieve sinus congestion, and soothe irritated mucous membranes.
- How to Use: Drink peppermint tea or inhale peppermint essential oil by adding a few drops to a bowl of hot water and inhaling the steam. You can also use peppermint-based chest rubs.

3. Ginger (Zingiber officinale)
- Benefits: Ginger has anti-inflammatory and antimicrobial properties that can help reduce nasal congestion and provide relief from sinus pressure.
- How to Use: Drink ginger tea or chew on fresh ginger slices. You can also inhale steam from ginger-infused hot water.

4. Garlic (Allium sativum)
- Benefits: Garlic has antimicrobial properties that can help fight off infections and reduce congestion in the sinuses.
- How to Use: Incorporate raw garlic into your meals or drink garlic tea by steeping crushed garlic cloves in hot water.

5. Turmeric (Curcuma longa)
- Benefits: Turmeric contains curcumin, which has anti-inflammatory properties that can help reduce inflammation in the sinuses and provide relief from congestion.
- How to Use: Add turmeric powder to your meals or drink turmeric tea by steeping turmeric powder in hot water.

6. Licorice Root (Glycyrrhiza glabra)
- Benefits: Licorice root has expectorant properties that can help thin mucus and promote sinus drainage, providing relief from congestion.

- How to Use: Drink licorice root tea or chew on licorice root sticks.

7. Elderberry (Sambucus nigra)
- Benefits: Elderberry has antiviral properties that can help fight off infections and reduce congestion in the sinuses.
- How to Use: Drink elderberry tea or take elderberry supplements according to the recommended dosage on the product label.

Important Considerations:
- Hydration: Drink plenty of fluids, such as water, herbal teas, and broths, to help thin mucus and promote sinus drainage.
- Steam Inhalation: Inhaling steam from hot water can help moisturize nasal passages, loosen mucus, and provide temporary relief from congestion.
- Rest and Humidity: Get plenty of rest and use a humidifier to add moisture to the air, which

www.ingramcontent.com/pod-product-compliance
Lightning Source LLC
Chambersburg PA
CBHW081211260726
48653CB00010BA/3602
* 9 7 9 8 3 2 7 1 6 1 6 7 2 *